BACK IN A HEART BEAT

To my darling Xav
Thankyou so much for your
efforts a your entertaining wid
You did a fantastic job at
Shock around the block
with much love from
Mum

09.10.15

BACK IN A HEART BEAT

Busting the myths about sudden cardiac arrest
and why bystanders can safely use defibrillators

ANNE HOLLAND

WRITING MATTERS PUBLISHING

Published by
Writing Matters Publishing (UK)
10 Lovelace Court
Bethersden Kent TN26 3AY
www.writingmatterspublishing.com
info@writingmatterspublishing.com

First published 2015

A Cataloguing-in-Publication record is available from the
National Library of Australia.

ISBN
978 0 9575440 5 5 (pbk)
978 0 9575440 6 2 (ebk–ePub)

Edited by Robyn Kent, RAK Editing Services
Designed and typeset by Helen Christie, Blue Wren Books
Graphics by Rebecca Mercer, Start Today Studio

defibfirst.com.au

urbanlifesavers.org.au

Proceeds from the sale of this book will be allocated
to not-for-profit Urban Lifesavers for development
of AED education programs.

'To live in the hearts we leave behind is not to die.'

THOMAS CAMPBELL

Dedicated to the memory of

Paul John 'Dutchy' Holland
(20 October 1951 – 17 February 2008) aged 56 years

My husband for 30 years and father of our five children,
Bridgette, Paul, Gerard, Xavier and Damien

Sudden cardiac arrest claimed Paul prematurely when he
still had so much more to do, to contribute and to enjoy

He would now be the proud father-in-law of David Lawes (Bridgette)
and Zoe Siskos (Paul) and adoring grandfather of
Samuel Paul Holland (2013), Edward Paul Lawes (2014) and
Maxwell Charles Holland (2015)

Paul was an honourable, hard-working, family man
who modelled his life on the following creed:

Leadership

A leader is best, when people barely know he exists
Not so good, when people obey and acclaim him
Worse, when they despise him
"Fail to honour people, they fail to honour you"
But of a good leader who talks little, when his work is done
and his aim fulfilled, they will say, "We did this ourselves."

LAO-TSE - *THE WAY OF LIFE ACCORDING TO LAO-TZU [SIC]:*
AN AMERICAN VERSION BY WITTER BYNNER

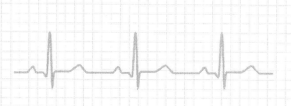

CONTENTS

Foreword   xi
Defibrillation brought me 'Back in a Heart Beat'   xiii
Preface   xv
Acknowledgements   xxi

Introduction   1

Part One
Automated external defibrillators and the workplace   9
 1 A case for providing AEDs in the workplace   11
 2 Incidence of cardiac arrest compared with other causes of death 16
 3 Roadblocks to providing AEDs in the workplace   23
 4 Industry adoption of AEDs   28
 5 Summary of workplace concerns and obligations   37

Part Two
Sudden cardiac arrest   41
 6 What is sudden cardiac arrest?   43
 7 Sudden cardiac arrest in young people   55
 8 The chain of survival   64

Part Three
The importance of defibrillation   71
 9 History of defibrillation to present day technology   73
10 How AEDs save lives   84
11 Public access defibrillation program   100
12 Why are education and training so important?   113

Part Four

Busting the myths about cardiac arrest and defibrillation   125

13   Myth 1 – Sudden cardiac arrest is a heart attack   127

14   Myth 2 – Rescuers can be sued for rendering first aid   134

15   Myth 3 – AEDs can shock someone who doesn't need
to be shocked   140

16   Myth 4 – An AED could cause further harm or injury
to the victim   149

17   Myth 5 – Paramedics will arrive in time   154

18   Myth 6 – Only qualified professionals can use an AED   161

19   Myth 7 – An AED in the workplace increases liability   169

Part Five

DRSABCD   185

20   Emergency Action Plan   187

21   Danger – hazards, risks, obstructions, safety issues   189

22   Response   194

23   Send for help   199

24   Airway   206

25   Check for breathing   210

26   Compressions   213

27   Defibrillation   227

Conclusion   246

About the author   253

Appendix A – Joint statement on early access to defibrillation   255

Appendix B – Governance of first aid training in Australia   263

Appendix C – Good Samaritan legislation in Australia   268

Appendix D – Australian Resuscitation Council Press Release 2006   270

Glossary   273

Notes   276

Bibliography   283

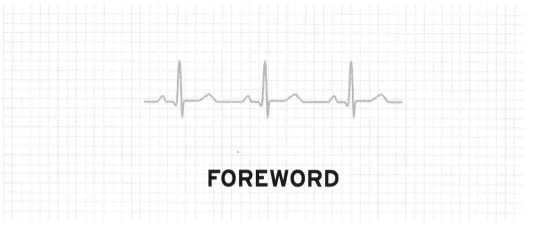

FOREWORD

Sudden Cardiac Arrest can happen anywhere and at any time. There is a 10% reduction in survival for every minute treatment is delayed and without early care the outcome can be poor.

Survival from cardiac arrest depends on a fully integrated system of care that combines early recognition that someone has collapsed and activation of the Emergency Medical Services system (000), early CPR, early access to defibrillation and early advanced care provided by paramedics and transport to hospital care.

Historically, early defibrillation required detailed knowledge of cardiac rhythms and was restricted to health professionals, however the development of Automated External Defibrillators, that can analyse heart rhythms and recommend a shock be delivered, has opened this life saving skill up to anyone with little or no training.

AEDs are relatively inexpensive, safe and simple to use. They are becoming increasingly available within workplaces, community locations, or as part of a formal Public Access Defibrillation (PAD) program, and allow lifesaving defibrillation to be delivered within minutes of a collapse occurring.

Victoria has some of the highest survival rates from cardiac arrest in the world and early CPR and early access defibrillation programs have played a critical role in this success. Bystander CPR rates for witnessed cardiac arrests have increased from 43% in 2004–05 to 75% in 2013–14 and there has been a 10-fold increase in the use of AEDs by members of the public for patients in shockable rhythms over the past decade (VACAR Annual Report 2013–14).

These statistics are comforting but we can't rest on our laurels and there is much more to do.

Anne has experienced firsthand the impact that cardiac arrest can have and I commend her vision and passion to increase the availability and knowledge of the use of AEDs in the community and to ultimately save more lives.

Associate Professor
Tony Walker ASM FPA
Chair, Victorian Branch,
Australian Resuscitation Council

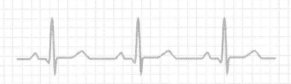

DEFIBRILLATION BROUGHT ME 'BACK IN A HEART BEAT'

I owe my job to Rupert Murdoch. But I owe my life to Kerry Packer, the media mogul who financed the rollout of "Packer-whackers" in NSW ambulances after a polo field heart attack almost killed him 25 years ago. Like Mr Packer, I was brought back to life by a defibrillator after I suffered a cardiac arrest a few months ago in a Sydney street. I told the story in The Australian, where I work as a science and higher education reporter.

The story paid tribute to the good Samaritan urban lifesavers who saved me – the ex-paramedic, registered nurse, flight attendant and others who recognised the situation as an emergency. They got me out of my car and applied CPR, keeping oxygenated blood flowing through my body until the ambulance arrived.

These wonderful people made my survival possible. But it was the defibrillator that saved my life by jolting my heart back into a viable rhythm. "We are having a defibrillator installed at home," a reader also named John announced in an online comment. "I will put a notice on our letterbox so everyone locally will know," said John, from the beachside suburb where I almost died. "We live on Rainbow Street, probably the steepest street in Sydney regularly used for wind sprints by local sports clubs. It may prove useful."

This is an understatement, and John should be applauded. Some 30,000 Australians suffer cardiac arrests every year, and about nine out of ten of them can't be revived. Those who can, usually experience significant brain and heart damage. I was extraordinarily lucky to escape this fate.

Ironically, my attack occurred straight across the road from a health centre. Amanda, one of my guardian angels, knew it probably had a defibrillator. But the place was locked up.

Contrast this with communities like Seattle, where defibrillators are accessible and ubiquitous, and people know how to use them. Some 65 per cent of cardiac arrest victims survive the experience in the Washington State port city, where defibrillation training is mandatory for university students and licensed drivers, among others.

Defibrillation is the low-hanging fruit of emergency medicine. Thousands of unnecessary deaths could be averted every year in Australia alone if people could get hold of defibrillators when they needed them, and knew what to do with them.

The latter part of this equation is pretty straightforward. Defibrillation machines are user-friendly, with robot voices explaining every step of the process.

People are understandably nervous about administering electric shocks to strangers. But the fact is, without your intervention, that stranger will almost certainly die. As with CPR, you can't make the situation any worse – a person experiencing cardiac arrest is already technically dead.

I am constantly reminded how lucky I am to still be here. But my story could be the norm rather than the exception. So many more of us – so many more husbands, wives, mothers, fathers, sons, daughters – could be Back in a Heart Beat. Let's work together to make that possibility a reality.

John Ross,
journalist,
The Australian

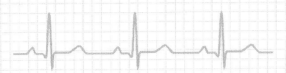

PREFACE

*'To every man there comes in his lifetime that special moment
when he is figuratively tapped on the shoulder and offered a chance
to do a very special thing, unique to him and fitted to his talents.
What a tragedy if that moment finds him unprepared or unqualified
for that which would be his finest hour.'*

APOCRYPHAL CHURCHILL

Urban lifesavers are ordinary people who take the extraordinary action to save the life of someone who has suffered a sudden cardiac arrest by quickly applying an automated external defibrillator (AED) without fear or hesitation.

Sudden cardiac arrest is the *one* cause of death for which any person, without any first aid or medical training, can actually restore the victim to life – but recovery is time critical. The many myths and misunderstandings that pervade folklore in the community and workplace prevent bystanders from taking those crucial lifesaving steps in time to make a difference.

Defibrillation is the only definitive first aid treatment for cardiac arrest and is the key to survival; however, the problem is there are too few publically accessible AEDs and too few people who have the knowledge and confidence to apply one.

We need to bust the myths and fears associated with the use of defibrillators by members of the public. You don't have to be a doctor or God to act and jolt someone back into life – an AED is all you need to make it happen. Anyone can do it with just a little knowledge!

After the myths are busted, the next step will be to influence legislative change so that AEDs become lawfully mandated and as commonplace as fire extinguishers in the workplace and community.

None of us are immune – sudden cardiac arrest happened in my family and it can happen in yours – to someone you love or even yourself. Sudden cardiac arrest can strike anyone – young or old, male or female. Survival depends on the time elapsed and the rapid response of bystander witnesses – regardless of their level of first aid training. There are varying estimates around the world but on average survival drops by 9%–10% for every minute that passes without defibrillation.

The missing link in the chain of survival is too often the AED.

An AED is intelligent; we just have to be trusting enough to let it do its *magic*!

Allow me to uncover the shocking truths about defibrillation and show you how to trust the AED and become an urban lifesaver.

This book has been written to be read in its entirety or as a resource with stand-alone chapters. Therefore there is some intentional repetition for the purpose of context, understanding and reinforcement.

The following chapters will discuss the intriguing history and technology of defibrillation, bust the myths and fears associated with public access AEDs, and explore the roadblocks and implications for widespread placement of AEDs in workplaces and public spaces.

Myth 1
Sudden cardiac arrest is a heart attack – there is nothing bystanders can do because it is too late or only doctors can diagnose and treat it.

Truth
Sudden cardiac arrest causes death but is not a heart attack. A cardiac arrest is an abnormality of the electrical system that stimulates the heart to beat. Although a cardiac arrest can be caused by a heart attack, there are multiple other causes affecting all age groups and both genders.

A heart attack is a blockage of an artery supplying blood to the heart muscle, that is, a plumbing abnormality. Sometimes a heart attack can result in a cardiac arrest; however, not everyone who has a heart attack has a cardiac arrest (dies). It is possible to survive a heart attack but it is not possible to survive a cardiac arrest without treatment with a defibrillator and anyone can apply an AED.

Myth 2
A rescuer who performs first aid and applies a defibrillator can be held liable and sued if the outcome of a cardiac arrest is not successful, that is, if the victim does not survive.

Truth
The law ('Good Samaritan' legislation) protects people who render first aid in good faith. First aid responders have never been and would not be held liable or be sued for applying a defibrillator while attempting to resuscitate a victim of cardiac arrest who is, in fact, already dead.

Myth 3
An AED can shock someone who doesn't need to be shocked.

Truth
An AED is designed to detect and analyse the electrical activity of the victim's heart. An AED must first be applied directly to the victim's bare chest and then will advise a shock *only* if it detects a lethal heart rhythm. An AED is safe and cannot be used inappropriately, nor can it shock the wrong person. It will not shock someone who does not need to be defibrillated, that is, it will not shock if it detects a normal heart rhythm.

Myth 4
An AED can cause harm or injury to the victim.

Truth
Someone who is in cardiac arrest is dead; therefore, it is not possible to injure them any further. An AED will do no harm because it will only work if it detects a life-threatening heart rhythm that requires a lifesaving shock. More harm is done to the victim by not rendering

aid and by not applying an AED to them because they have almost no chance of survival without early defibrillation and cardiopulmonary resuscitation (CPR).

Myth 5

An AED is not needed because all that rescuers need to do is phone Triple Zero (000) and an ambulance will arrive with a defibrillator, or there will be enough time to get the casualty to a nearby hospital.

Truth

Any delay in applying a defibrillator dramatically reduces the victim's chance of survival. Average ambulance response times in Australia are often more than 10 minutes but an AED needs to be applied within the first five minutes for the greatest chance of survival. There is also no time to get a victim of cardiac arrest to hospital regardless of how close the hospital is. Ambulance Victoria 2014 statistics reveal that cardiac arrest victims who are defibrillated by witnesses are three times more likely to survive in the long term than those victims who are not defibrillated until paramedics or medical aid arrive.

Myth 6

Only medical professionals, paramedics, or first aid–trained persons can use an AED.

Truth

Sudden cardiac arrest is the one cause of death that bystanders can actually reverse if they apply an AED quickly. Anyone, regardless of their level of training, can safely and effectively apply an AED to someone who is in cardiac arrest. The key to survival is immediate CPR and – most importantly – early defibrillation. An AED is automated and will only work if necessary after it detects a lethal heart rhythm. All that a rescuer needs to do is apply the pads and let the AED do the rest.

Myth 7

An AED in the workplace increases liability risks for the employer and gives the impression that the workplace is stressful and unsafe for employees, if an AED is needed to be on standby.

Truth

An AED is the most vital piece of emergency first aid equipment and the only effective treatment for cardiac arrest. Therefore, having an AED in the workplace increases safety and peace of mind and decreases workplace risk and liability. Workplaces are in breach of occupational health and safety (OH&S) laws if they do not have fire extinguishers and evacuation plans. Having a fire extinguisher on site is a form of insurance and does not mean that a workplace is more likely to have a fire thereby making the workplace unsafe.

The same argument applies to an AED – it is form of insurance and provides an effective remedy if the emergency event occurs. Having an AED on the premises reduces the risk of liability because the AED enables first aid officers to perform the lifesaving skills for which they have been trained and minimises the risk of an unsuccessful outcome, that is, death.

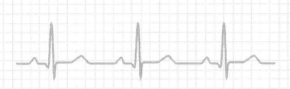

ACKNOWLEDGEMENTS

'If you don't make a difference in life, it is a waste of a life.'

GLENN NICHOLSON

The raw grief and devastation that my children, Bridgette, Paul, Gerard, Xavier and Damien suffered following the sudden loss of their Dad was harrowing to watch. I felt so powerless to help them and it will haunt me forever. Now I hope that my commitment to raise awareness about the importance of bystanders becoming urban lifesavers by taking action during a cardiac arrest will ease their pain a little with the establishment of a lasting legacy in Paul's memory.

In 2014, following Gerard's recommendation, I registered for the Key Person of Influence (KPI) program in Melbourne. KPI is a 40-week business and leadership development program for entrepreneurs who have a vision and a passion to expand their ideas and businesses. Without the KPI program:

- This book would not have been written.
- The public awareness campaign to educate ordinary people on how to become an urban lifesaver by applying an AED to a victim of cardiac arrest may not have become a reality.
- The not-for-profit Urban Lifesavers organisation would not exist.
- The fundraising function 'Shock around the Clock' during 'Shocktober' – sudden cardiac arrest awareness month – would not have been born.

At the end of the program in December 2014, I was privileged to win the KPI pitching competition 'PitchFest' and was awarded the first ever, in Australia, perfect score of 10 from all four judges. As a mature aged woman with an over-abundance of self-doubt and without significant business acumen, no-one was more surprised with that result than me. Self-praise is no recommendation, however, that success was a pivotal turning point in my aspirations because it gave me a much needed boost in self-belief and sense of relevance; reinforced the validation of my message and inspired me to just get it done. In KPI vernacular, this is referred to as GSD – Get S✱✱t Done!

I thank the creators of the KPI program, Daniel Priestley and Glen Carlson, for their brainchild. The KPI program was nominated in *The Huffington Post* in 2014 as the number one entrepreneurial leadership program in the world and has significantly changed the lives of KPI alumni.

I also wish to express my gratitude to the following people for their support and advice:

My friend and colleague – Frances Nugent for her patient review of my manuscript
Foreword – Assoc. Professor Tony Walker ASM
KPI publishing mentors – Andrew Griffiths and Andrew Priestley
Book designer – Helen Christie, Blue Wren Books
Editor – Robyn Kent, RAK Editing Services
Marketing lateral thinker – Adrian Jobson, AltusQ
Graphic designer – Rebecca Mercer, Start Today Studio
Printer and friend – Frank Cariss
Generous contributors – Geoff Allen, Angela Bourke, Sue and Ashlea Buckman, Glen Burgin, Leigh Clarnette, Jason Cripps, Jon Delaney, Leigh and Megan Fotheringham, Jenny Gifford, Chris and Maria Hogan, Kaydee Horne, Karen Howden-Clarnette, Samantha Jobe, Janelle Mitchell, Sean Purcell, Kevin Rizzoli, John Ross, Tara Smith, Michael Stapleton, Michael Sukkar, Jenny Whiteford.

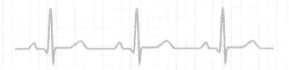

INTRODUCTION

'When we least expect it, life sets us a challenge to test our courage and willingness to change; at such a moment, there is no point in pretending that nothing has happened or in saying that we are not yet ready. The challenge will not wait. Life does not look back ...'

PAULO COELHO

Five pieces of luck

On the day that he died in 2009, Jon Delaney was a lucky man five times over. Two weeks after his fortieth birthday, Jon was busy at work. He had things to do. A family man and a businessman with a high-flying corporate lifestyle, Jon didn't have time to stop – *until his heart did!*

Jon, just 40, had suffered a heart attack. His first bit of luck was that his heart did not stop beating immediately. Although he experienced some warning signs and symptoms – chest pain and feeling unwell and sweaty – he initially ignored them. He had work to do and phone calls to make – he'd go to the doctor later.

His second bit of luck was the insistence of a work colleague that he be driven to hospital without any further delay.

His third bit of luck was that he did not go into cardiac arrest in the car. If a driver suddenly stops in traffic and tries to perform cardio-pulmonary resuscitation (CPR) on a casualty – who is seated in an upright position and wearing a seatbelt, with no control of the casualty's airway – while also phoning for help, the situation is not going to end well. Just removing the casualty from the vehicle takes vital minutes.

That delay dramatically reduces the cardiac arrest victim's chances of survival.

Jon's fourth bit of luck was that he made it to hospital – where it seemed his luck had run out. Jon suffered a sudden cardiac arrest on arrival in the emergency department and he 'died'.

Luck, however, was still on Jon's side. His final and most important stroke of luck was that he had made it to a hospital before his heart went into cardiac arrest and emergency medical assistance was immediately available to save him. He was quickly defibrillated in the emergency department and revived.

Had Jon suffered his cardiac arrest at work, he more than likely would not have survived because his workplace did not have an automated external defibrillator (AED) on the premises. His life was saved by the quick thinking and insistence of his colleague and by reaching the hospital emergency department in time.

As happened to my husband, many people who suffer a sudden cardiac arrest get no warning and literally 'drop dead' on the spot. A sudden cardiac arrest means that the victim is deceased and needs rapid defibrillation to restore a normal heart rhythm. Without an AED, a rescuer can still perform CPR at the scene while waiting for paramedics to arrive with a defibrillator. This would prolong survival and give the victim a chance but, more often than not, there would not be a happy ending.

Jon made the near-fatal mistake of not taking his symptoms seriously and he delayed getting help until he finished important tasks that needed his attention. Those tasks would never have been completed if some good fortune had not been on his side!

Today, over five years later, Jon is indeed a very lucky man. He recovered from his cardiac arrest and is still a family man and businessman but he has a very different approach to his life and lifestyle. He is also a strong supporter of AEDs in all workplaces because he is living proof that early defibrillation and early access to emergency medical care can save lives.

Sudden cardiac arrest

What is it and who does it affect?

Sudden cardiac arrest (SCA) occurs when the heart's electrical control system suddenly stops the heart beating or pumping blood. Sudden cardiac arrest strikes an estimated 33,000 Australians each year. Cardiovascular (heart and blood vessels) disease (CVD) is the leading cause of death in the industrialised world but there is widespread lack of awareness of its incidence and significance. Cardiac arrest does not discriminate – it strikes males and females, young and old, and can strike anyone, of any age, anytime, anywhere. SCA has no warning signs and 75% (three-quarters) of cardiac arrests will occur outside of a hospital, that is, in the community and workplace. Therefore it is critical that bystanders react promptly by starting CPR and applying an AED to give the casualty the best chance of survival.

CASE STUDY: Sean Purcell's story of survival on a Victorian beach

Another very lucky man who should be dead is Sean Purcell. In July 2014, 37 year old Sean suffered a sudden cardiac arrest while jogging on Whites Beach at Torquay in Victoria. Unlike Jon, Sean did not have a heart attack. He had a viral lung infection which affected his heart and caused it to stop beating; he dropped face first into the water. Unlike Jon, he was not near a hospital or any medical aid.

Sean's life was saved by nine quick-thinking strangers who dragged him from the water and kept him alive for 25 minutes by taking turns to perform CPR. They also had the presence of mind to locate a defibrillator at a nearby golf course and they used it to restore his heart rhythm. One rescuer had to jog 1.5 km and back on sand to deliver the AED to Sean's side.

The tide was coming in and the coastal terrain was rugged. Sean's team of urban lifesavers needed to move his body several times up the beach, away from the rising tide. Twenty minutes after he arrested, the paramedics arrived; however, the beach vegetation and sand dunes made access very difficult. The medical helicopter was unable to land on the beach and his rescuers had to carry him up through the dunes to the waiting chopper.

Sean was air lifted to Geelong Hospital where he was placed in an induced coma for five days. His wife, Kelly, and family were told his prognosis was bleak and that 'if' he woke up, he would be suffering high-end brain damage. But Sean did survive and he thrived. A year later, because of the efforts of strangers, Sean has recovered with 100% brain function and he is back working full-time. He has an implanted defibrillator which recently discharged an internal shock, when his heart went into an unsafe rhythm, and saved his life yet again. He has been given a second chance and is committed to sharing his story in order to shed a light on the importance of CPR training and accessibility to public defibrillators.

Jon's and Sean's stories both ended with the best possible outcomes. Without early implementation of CPR and defibrillation, SCA would have had very different and tragic consequences for their wives and children. Sadly, my husband Paul (a father of five) did not survive because he did not have early access to CPR, defibrillation and emergency medical care – no-one witnessed his cardiac arrest and we did not find him in time to be able to help him.

Is sudden cardiac arrest the same as a heart attack?

Although Jon and my husband, Paul, both suffered heart attacks that precipitated cardiac arrests, Sean's cardiac arrest was caused by a virus. A heart attack is a separate event from a cardiac arrest. Suffering a heart attack does not automatically mean that a SCA will occur. However, the likelihood of a cardiac arrest resulting from a heart attack is extremely high. No-one experiencing symptoms of a heart attack should delay seeking medical attention because there is a very great risk that they may go into cardiac arrest without warning. The difference between cardiac arrest and heart attack is described in further detail in Chapter 13 'Myth 1 – Sudden cardiac arrest is a heart attack'.

Leading cause of death in the world

Cardiovascular disease (CVD) refers to all diseases and conditions involving the heart and blood vessels. Health data compiled from more than 190 countries show that CVD remains the number one cause of death in the world with 17.3 million deaths each year, according to the American Heart Association. That number is expected to rise to more than 23.6 million by 2030.

CVD is the leading cause of death in Australia and affects one in six Australians (3.72 million people or two out of three families). The main types of CVD in Australia are coronary artery disease, stroke, and heart failure/cardiomyopathy. These diseases are disabling and prevent 1.4 million people from living a full life. According to Australian heart disease statistics, analysed by the Australian Bureau of Statistics (ABS), CVD claimed the lives of 43,603 Australians in 2013, deaths which were largely preventable. On average, one Australian dies as a result of CVD every 12 minutes.[1]

Although the number of deaths from CVD fell by 13.3% between 2002 and 2013 (from 50,294 to 43,603), CVD still accounted for nearly 30% of all deaths in Australia in 2013. CVD is one of Australia's largest health problems. Despite improvements over the last few decades, it remains the most expensive disease group in Australia and is one of the biggest burdens on the national economy, costing billions of dollars.[2]

In a press release on 16 December 2014, National CEO of the Heart Foundation of Australia, Mary Barry, said:

> The *Australian heart disease statistics 2014* inaugural compendium provides some worrying statistics about the changing nature of Australia's leading killer – cardiovascular disease.

> Cardiovascular disease remains the biggest killer of Australians and is the most expensive disease to treat nationally. Unfortunately, with it accounting for 11% of direct healthcare expenditure, it remains a national health priority in name only. Unlike other health priorities, there is no nationally funded action plan to drive improvements in prevention, early detection and management of cardiovascular disease.[3]

Comparison with other causes of death

SCA is a leading cause of death among adults over the age of 40 in the United States and other countries. According to the Sudden Cardiac Arrest Foundation, the number of people who die each year from SCA is roughly equivalent to the number of deaths from Alzheimer's disease, assault with firearms, breast cancer, cervical cancer, colorectal cancer, diabetes, HIV, house fires, motor vehicle accidents, prostate cancer and suicides combined. SCA is a life-threatening condition – but it can be treated successfully through early intervention with cardiopulmonary resuscitation (CPR), defibrillation, advanced cardiac life support, and mild therapeutic hypothermia (lowering of body temperature).[4]

CVD is the most common killer of women, who have caught up with men in the incidence of cardiac disease. It kills more men than prostate cancer and more women than breast cancer. Coronary artery disease, which causes heart attacks, kills 55 Australians each day (one Australian every 26 minutes).

Dr Lyn Roberts, former CEO of the National Heart Foundation of Australia, said in a media release on 1 June 2013:

> Many people are still surprised to learn that heart disease is the number one killer of Australian women and that it claims more than three times as many female lives as breast cancer. We're very concerned that three in five women do not recognise heart disease as a serious female health issue.[5]

Survival rates – out-of-hospital cardiac arrest

It is estimated that over 325,000 out-of-hospital cardiac arrests (OHCA) are attended by emergency medical services (EMS) each year in the United States. In cases where a public access AED is applied at the scene by bystanders, the long-term survival rate is three times greater than those who are defibrillated after arrival of EMS. These trends are similar to Australian survival rates following the application of an AED by urban lifesaver witnesses.

The only definitive first aid treatment for victims of SCA is defibrillation. SCA happens without warning and the majority of people have no previously recognised symptoms of heart disease. For the best chance of survival from SCA caused by a shockable rhythm, an AED should ideally be used within the first three to five minutes after collapse. Currently less than 5% of all victims of SCA survive, largely because a defibrillator does not arrive in time. Prompt use of an AED can dramatically increase the survival rate to over 80%.

Increasing access to AEDs

There are multiple causes of cardiac arrest and in the same way that seatbelts and air bags cannot prevent death in every road trauma casualty, AEDs will not save every victim of cardiac arrest. However, thousands of lives could be restored if ordinary people had immediate access to an AED.

It is well established that if early defibrillation or bystander-initiated resuscitation efforts are not implemented, it is rare for the victim to survive. 'The automated external defibrillator (AED) has been described as the single most important development in the treatment of SCA. These devices are now widely available and increasingly used by people, often with little or no training, to re-start the heart of a victim of SCA'.[6] When an AED is applied soon after a cardiac arrest, the majority of victims can survive.

The primary goals of this book are education and raising awareness about the importance of public access defibrillation. The ultimate objective is to achieve legislative change so that AEDs become an essential and compulsory component of first aid kits throughout the country.

Until legislative change becomes a reality, the most pressing problem is to debunk the mythology surrounding AEDs so that bystanders are more willing and confident to 'have a go' and jolt someone back into life following a SCA.

The myths about AEDs include:
1. Sudden cardiac arrest is a heart attack and only doctors can diagnose and treat it.
2. A rescuer who applies a defibrillator can be held liable and sued if the victim does not survive.
3. An AED can shock someone who doesn't need to be shocked.
4. An AED can cause harm or injury to the victim.
5. An AED isn't needed because all the rescuers need to do is phone emergency services and paramedics will arrive with a defibrillator, or there will be enough time to get the casualty to a hospital.

6. Only medical professionals, paramedics and first aid-trained persons can use an AED.
7. An AED in the workplace increases liability risks for the employer.

Because of these myths, layperson bystanders often believe that it is too late because the victim is dead and there is nothing they can do except wait for more qualified responders to arrive.

The chapters to follow will bust the myths surrounding AEDs, and will increase knowledge and awareness of the critical role that bystander CPR and public access AEDs play in saving lives in the community. Everyone should aspire to be an urban lifesaver. You never know when you or someone you love will need a hero who knows how to use an AED.

Part One

AUTOMATED EXTERNAL DEFIBRILLATORS AND THE WORKPLACE

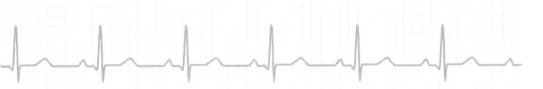

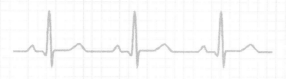

CHAPTER 1

A CASE FOR PROVIDING AEDS IN THE WORKPLACE

*'You must remember that some things legally right
are not morally right.'*

ABRAHAM LINCOLN

Safety is increasingly becoming a core value in corporate mission statements. There is a duty of care incumbent upon employers and government agencies to provide the safest environment possible for their employees and customers. Large organisations (private and government) can have hundreds and even thousands of members of the general public entering their premises every day.

The 2012 *Joint statement on early access to defibrillation*, issued by St John Ambulance Australia, the Australian Resuscitation Council and the National Heart Foundation of Australia, noted that over 30,000 cases of sudden cardiac arrest occur within Australia each year. It reinforced the importance of raising public awareness that a prompt response to sudden cardiac arrest (SCA) is vital. A SCA is eminently treatable with prompt cardiopulmonary resuscitation (CPR) and early defibrillation but the chance of survival decreases by 9%–10% for every minute that defibrillation is delayed. Not enough has changed and too many avoidable deaths are still occurring since the joint statement declared three years ago that:

> Early access to defibrillation (EAD) for sudden cardiac arrest is a vital link in the universally recognised 'chain of survival,' as the time taken to defibrillation is a key predictor of survival. Within Australia, the concept of lay persons having access to and using automated external

defibrillators (AEDs) for out-of-hospital sudden cardiac arrest has gained increasing support as a result of its effectiveness in saving lives … However, more can be achieved by taking a systematic approach to the implementation of AED in the community providing greater access to and use of these devices for cardiac arrest. (Appendix A)

Regulatory changes in first aid training affecting the workplace

First aid training is a series of regulated units of competency within the Health Training Package (HLT) which is governed by the Community Services and Health Industry Skills Council and is regulated under the auspices of the Australian Government.

Until 2013 in Australia, an employer with 10 or more employees was required to provide first aid-trained personnel who were competent in performing CPR until paramedics arrived and took over. At that time, the regulations for the first aid unit of competency 'HLTCPR211A – Perform CPR' required the training participant to 'have an understanding' of what an AED was and how it worked. The unit of competency did not include mandatory training and assessment in the application of an AED during a cardiac arrest nor did an AED need to be available during training for participants to observe how it worked.

On July 1 2013 the Australian Resuscitation Council guidelines for first aid training were superseded and revised requirements were introduced to satisfy the key criteria. The CPR unit of competency was amended and renamed 'HLTAID001 – Provide cardiopulmonary resuscitation'. HLTAID001 has a new key element that requires training participants to be assessed and deemed competent in not only the performance of effective CPR but also in the application of an AED. For participants to be assessed as competent, the training provider must have AED training equipment available for practical demonstration and participants must demonstrate their ability to operate it. The new guidelines came into force on 1 July 2014, and all first aid personnel must complete that unit each year. Governance of first aid training is described in more detail in Appendix B.

Many workplaces have voluntarily installed AEDs; however, there is still significant resistance from employers to providing these lifesaving devices. Chapter 19, 'Myth 7 – An AED in the workplace increases liability' covers these inhibitors in more detail.

Implications for business

Although the Australian Government now requires that first aid personnel achieve competency in defibrillation, the government has not legislated that AEDs be mandatory inclusions in all first aid kits. The argument could be made that AEDs should be an essential inclusion in first aid kits in the workplace because if an incident happened where a defibrillator was required to carry out the first aid management of the casualty, the first aid officers could not perform the duties for which they had been trained if the device was not available.

Defibrillation must be provided in less than five minutes after cardiac arrest to give the victim the greatest likelihood of surviving and making a full, long-term recovery, that is, the victim returns to work and resumes normal life activities. After eight minutes without defibrillation, the victim could possibly be revived but the chances of success and a full recovery are slim. Having a defibrillator readily available could well mean the difference between life and death.

Duty of care

Businesses need to consider the duty of care implications when employers do not provide the very piece of equipment which they have trained their staff to use and which could actually save a life if someone had a cardiac arrest on the premises.

Businesses should also consider how the changes in first aid training regulations affect safety, risk, liability, governance and compliance for the employer and government agencies, not just for staff but also for customers and clients on their premises.

Cost of employee death, illness or injury

When an employee dies or suffers serious illness or injury, there is significant loss to industry in terms of lost time injury, productivity, replacement and training of personnel, sick-leave and termination payouts and, potentially, liability and compliance costs. The unexpected death of a colleague at work results in very significant psychological and emotional shock for other staff, which imposes additional burden on the business. The Australian Bureau of Statistics (ABS) estimates that the years of potential life lost (YPLL) from cardiac causes of death in Australia is more than 110,000 years.[7] Having an AED in the workplace or available in the community could save thousands of lives each year.

CASE STUDY: Mr Michael Sukkar, MP

The Federal Member for Deakin, Mr Michael Sukkar MP, suffered a sudden cardiac arrest while playing basketball in Nunawading, Victoria, in 2008. He was 26 years of age at the time and he is one of the very lucky ones who survived, due to two pieces of good luck.

Luckily for Michael, a nurse and a doctor witnessed his collapse and started CPR immediately. Even more incredibly, paramedic Andrew Burns, who was 200 metres away at the Metropolitan Ambulance Service communications centre, intercepted the Triple Zero (000) (EMS) call and was courtside minutes later with a defibrillator.

Andrew knew when he heard that call that he could help Michael before any dispatch unit could arrive. 'I knew no one else could beat me there, so I was here within minutes,' Mr Burns said. 'As a paramedic you get a lot of wins and losses, but this was the pinnacle, being able to bring back a young man.'

Following Michael's cardiac arrest he had an implanted defibrillator inserted, which has never been activated. What is known is that although his heart stopped beating, he did not have a heart attack as most people assume (see Chapter 13 'Myth 1 - Sudden cardiac arrest is a heart attack').

Michael, who is now fighting fit and happily married, has gone on to serve in the Parliament of Australia as the Member for the Deakin electorate in Melbourne's eastern suburbs.

He believes the incident may have inspired him to move from law into politics. 'When I was elected, a lot of people asked me what motivated me to get into politics,' he said. 'On reflection, while I wasn't conscious of it, I think this was a defining experience.'

The basketball stadium where Michael played is now fitted with an AED, and Andrew believes it is important that people in the community have access to AEDs in emergency situations.

Michael believes that without an accessible defibrillator, he would not have survived and gone onto to become a family man and give back to his community. Mr Michael Sukkar MP is an advocate of public access defibrillation programs.

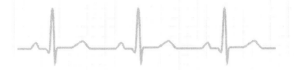

CHAPTER 2

INCIDENCE OF CARDIAC ARREST COMPARED WITH OTHER CAUSES OF DEATH

'The purpose of life is to matter – to count, to stand for something, to have it make some difference that we lived at all.'

LEO ROSTEN

Road fatalities

Problem
Road crashes are a major cause of death and injury in Australia. The annual cost of road crashes is estimated to be more than A$15 billion.

There was community outrage in the Australian state of Victoria in 1969 when the number of road deaths for the year reached 1,034, prompting the media and the police to 'Declare War on 1034'. The following year, 1970, Victoria had its worst ever road toll: 1,061. According to the Australian Bureau of Statistics (ABS), the national road toll in 1970 was 3,798, representing 30.4 fatalities per 100,000 persons.[8]

Action
This number of fatalities and the impact these deaths had on families and the community was rightly considered untenable and since that time enormous amounts of money and manpower have been expended on mass public education and advertising campaigns; a crackdown on speeding and drink driving with the introduction of breath testing, (and more recently drug testing), reduced speed limits, speed cameras and enforcement of penalties; the introduction of compulsory seatbelts

and motorcycle helmets; safer cars; improved driver education; stricter learner conditions; and better roads, all of which resulted in dramatic reductions in road trauma.

Result
In 2014, 249 road fatalities were recorded in Victoria (242 in 2013). Australia-wide, 1,156 fatalities were recorded in 2014 (1,193 in 2013). The 2014 road toll represented 4.9 fatalities per 100,000 persons – the lowest figure on record and about one-sixth of the national fatality rate in 1970. Improvements to roads and vehicles, enactment of road safety legislation, intensive public education and enhanced police enforcement technology have all contributed to the turnaround in the road toll.[9] Similar campaigns are now in place to reduce risks to cyclists and pedestrians.

Comparison with sudden cardiac arrest
Compare these statistics for road fatalities with the estimated 6,000 out-of-hospital cardiac arrests (OHCA) attended by Ambulance Victoria each year and approximately 33,000 OHCAs nationwide. SCA is the one cause of death for which the ordinary person can actually restore a victim to life. All that is needed is to provide public access defibrillators and educate laypersons on how to use them. Unlike the efforts made to reduce the number of road fatalities, there are no comparable or targeted public awareness campaigns, legislation or funding for establishing public access defibrillation (PAD) programs.

Fire- and smoke-related fatalities

Problem
There were 258 fire-related fatalities in England in 2014–15,[10] compared with the British Heart Foundation estimate of 60,000 cardiac arrests each year.[11] These figures show that a person in England is 233 times more likely to have a cardiac arrest than to die in a fire and yet fire extinguishers are compulsory (in workplaces and all locations where members of the public gather) but defibrillators are not.

In Australia, the latest ABS listings for causes of death (updated March 2015), show that cardiac-related conditions (including 33,000 cardiac arrests) are the cause of about 44,000 Australian deaths each year, compared with 56 fatalities in 2013 attributed to exposure from fire, smoke and heat.[12]

Action
Australian Standard 2444, governed by regulations for the Building Code of Australia, requires that at least one fire extinguisher is located in commercial premises or public meeting places. For example, there are extinguishers for Class A (paper, wood, textiles) and Class E (electrical) fires. For Class A fires, extinguishers must be accessible every 15 walkable metres and for Class E fires, every 20 walkable metres.[13]

Depending on the size of a building and the products stored within, a combination of as many as six different types of portable fire extinguishers may be required to cover a variety of fire situations. Owners/occupiers of buildings are also required to provide evidence that fire equipment has been supplied and/or maintained in accordance with relevant Australian Standards. Insurance companies may also require evidence that regular maintenance has been carried out.

There are no specific requirements for fire extinguishers in private dwellings; however, since 1995, Australian legislation has required smoke detector alarms (hard wired to mains electricity and fitted with a battery backup) to be installed in all new residences and residences under renovation. Smoke detector alarms are also required by most states and territories to be retrospectively installed in residences.[14]

Result
Mandatory fire safety equipment in all range of buildings in Australia has resulted in a significant reduction in death, injury and property damage in the workplace, community and private residences.

Comparison with sudden cardiac arrest
The ABS registers deaths only and does not include the number of cardiac arrest victims who are revived. It is estimated that there are 33,000 sudden cardiac arrests (SCA) in Australia each year and 75%

occur outside of a hospital. The likelihood of suffering a SCA is about 590 times greater than the chance of dying in a fire-related incident. Yet workplaces must have fire extinguishers but not AEDs. The math doesn't add up and the law needs to respond accordingly.

Heart disease is one of the most common causes of death in the United Kingdom with the worst heart attack rate in Scotland. In an article published in *The Edinburgh Evening News*, 30 July 2014, Bryan Finlay, the Scottish Ambulance Service's community resuscitation development officer, said that:

> You're more likely to die of a cause related to heart disease than you are in a fire ... Do people generally know how to use a fire extinguisher? Not really, but they'll have a go if they need to. That's where we're trying to get to with defibrillators.[15]

Rescuers need to be able to find an AED in an emergency, but they are not in every building, unlike fire extinguishers. According to Mr Finlay:

> The issue is that there aren't that many defibrillators anywhere, so people don't go and look for them. What we need people to do is recognise the need for them, and hopefully one day, every place will have one.
>
> As far as I'm concerned, every new public building should have one. If you're encouraging people to come to your facility, you need to safeguard them ... (AEDs) should be in central locations, and clearly signposted ... many are locked away in cupboards and boxes by owners worried they might be stolen, rendering them effectively useless. We don't want the defibrillation to be delayed by seconds, because those seconds add up to be minutes. Time is against you.[16]

Declan O'Mahoney, CEO of HeartSine said that governments put millions into fire safety, prevention and training every year:

> We adapt buildings, put in emergency exits, invest in training and maintain fire extinguishers. If the same effort went into dealing with sudden cardiac arrest, we could help offset a significant number of deaths every year.[17]

The late Professor Ian Jacobs, who tragically died suddenly of a brain haemorrhage on 19 October 2014, was chair of the Australian Resuscitation Council (ARC) and co-chair of the International Liaison Committee on Resuscitation (ILCOR), and was strongly of the view that

AEDs should be mandatory equipment, similar to the provision of fire extinguishers in the workplace and public spaces.

Prostate, breast and skin cancer fatalities

Problem
In Australia in 2013, there were 3,112 deaths attributed to prostate cancer, 2,892 deaths attributed to breast cancer and 2,209 deaths caused by skin cancer (including melanoma).

Action
In conjunction with increased government spending on education, screening, research and treatment, there has been phenomenal success with public awareness and fund raising campaigns in Australia about prostate, breast and skin cancer.

Result
Fundraising campaigns have facilitated amazing progress in research, early detection, development of treatments and improved survivability. These developments, along with government-funded education and screening programs, have led to dramatic improvements in morbidity and mortality rates.

The breast cancer awareness foundations and networks in Australia are examples of outstanding successful programs. The impact of the Pink Lady 'Field of Women' on the Melbourne Cricket Ground once a year, where the field is covered with people wearing pink and filling the outline of a woman, has iconic status. The McGrath Foundation Pink Stumps Day during the Summer Cricket Series is another example of how breast cancer awareness has changed public perception, raised the profile of breast cancer and brought about very significant improvement with many lives saved.

The success of this campaign is as it should be – breast cancer is a major killer, particularly of women, in Australia and around the world. However, the number of people who suffer a SCA in Australia (estimated 33,000) is double the number of those diagnosed with breast cancer (15,740 projected for 2015) each year.[18]

The success of all of these campaigns should be acclaimed because prostate and breast cancers are major killers and Australia has the highest per capita incidence of skin cancer in the world.

Comparison with sudden cardiac arrest

The number of people who suffer a SCA is 11 times greater than the numbers who die from either prostate or breast cancer. SCA is 15 times more common than deaths resulting from skin cancer.[19]

SCA strikes more people than all cancers combined, yet there is no government funding for public access defibrillation (PAD) programs, nor is there anywhere near the level of awareness, action or public participation needed to find a remedy for this problem. A remedy that is already effective and available is the AED – it just needs to be implemented.

Treatment for cancer relies on specialist medical expertise; however, treatment of a cardiac arrest depends on the person standing next to the victim taking immediate action. Medical treatment later is of no use if the victim does not survive the cardiac arrest.

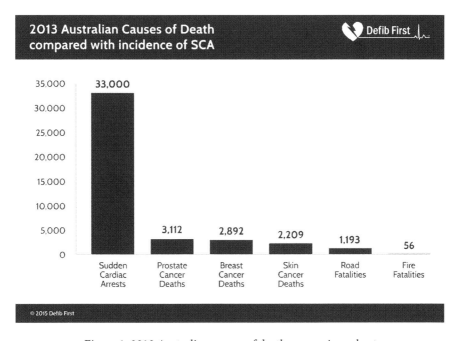

Figure 1. 2013 Australian causes of death comparison chart

Summary

It cannot be stressed enough that the arguments in this book for greater awareness and spending on public access AEDs and increased training on how to use them are not criticisms of expenditure on other health and safety campaigns. The arguments contained herein are for AED availability and public education and training to become commensurate with other public health initiatives, not to detract from them.

Figure 1 clearly shows that, of the major causes of death in Australia (sourced from the Australian Bureau of Statistics), cardiac arrest has the greatest impact on the population today. Despite cardiac arrest being the one cause of death that bystanders can actually reverse before medical assistance arrives, AEDs are not mandatory in the workplace and in the community. Why is there not more outrage and proactive campaigning on this issue?

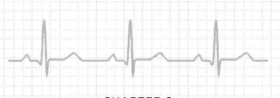

CHAPTER 3

ROADBLOCKS TO PROVIDING AEDS IN THE WORKPLACE

'The saddest aspect of life right now is that science gathers knowledge faster than society gathers wisdom.'

ISAAC ASIMOV

Attitudes to AEDs

Across the community, and particularly in the workplace, there is significant misunderstanding of sudden cardiac arrest: what it is, who it affects, and the role of defibrillation in saving the life of someone who is in cardiac arrest. Education programs are needed to uncover the truths and facts about AEDs and to dispel people's fears. Busting those myths and misunderstandings through education is the only way to encourage more people, regardless of whether they have first aid training, to 'have a go' and apply an automated external defibrillator (AED) without hesitation.

The same attitudes to AEDs prevail around the world. In an article, 'Learn how to use defibrillator and save lives', published in *The Edinburgh Evening News* on 30 July 2014, Paris Gourtsoyannis described how:

> Without really noticing it, every day we're surrounded by kits that can help keep us safe if the worst should happen. Burn your toast in the morning, and it will probably set off the smoke alarm. At your office or workplace, you're never far from the nearest fire extinguisher, and you may have a designated first-aider or fire warden. You probably know where the first aid kit is at home, even if it's at the back of the drawer, and you may have a carbon monoxide detector, too. But what about a device that could save your life if you had a heart attack [cardiac arrest]?

While fire extinguishers are required everywhere, most paramedics and firefighters will tell you they've used an AED far more often than a fire extinguisher.

Is failure to provide an AED comparable with a failure to have fire extinguishers on site as a safety precaution in case a fire breaks out? Failure to provide a fire extinguisher and evacuation plan would be a breach of occupational health and safety/workplace health and safety (OH&S/WHS) laws and the employer would be liable. Shouldn't the same onus of responsibility apply to providing an AED which is the only definitive treatment for sudden cardiac arrest (SCA)?

Liability issues

Is there potential for the organisation (public or private) to be held liable and to be sued if a casualty dies because first aid officers are trained to use an AED but a defibrillator is not available and so they cannot provide the most effective resuscitation treatment for a cardiac arrest?

While a successful liability lawsuit for not having an AED may seem unlikely under current Australian OH&S laws, people (both employees and customers) have a far greater awareness than ever before of their rights in the workplace, and businesses that do not move with the changes in training regulations may potentially be vulnerable.

There is a common perception that businesses are at a greater liability risk by having an AED on the premises (see Chapter 19 'Myth 7 – An AED in the workplace increases liability'), when in fact their liability is more likely to be decreased by providing an AED. Modern AEDs cannot be used inappropriately and it is not possible to do any further harm to a cardiac arrest victim who is, in effect, dead and will remain so unless defibrillated.

Costs

Purchase price
Businesses spend extraordinary amounts of money on technology, CCTV, security systems, fire equipment, evacuation drills and training to protect staff and property.

Perceptions about cost often create resistance to purchasing an AED. In Australia, the cost of an AED ranges between $2,000 and $3,000. AEDs have 7 to 10 year warranties, and come with long-life non-rechargeable batteries that last several years. The purchase price amortised over a conservative 10-year life of the device equates to only $200–$300 per year compared with the potential cost of a life lost. The increase in safety awareness and compliance and the reduction in liability should be a worthy and reasonable trade-off for the modest cost.

Two to three hundred dollars per year is not an excessive outlay compared with the significant loss to industry in relation to safety, productivity, lost time injury, replacing and training personnel, termination/sick-leave payouts, life insurance payments and, potentially, liability and compliance costs. Not to forget the potential for a civil liability law suit.

Cost of death or injury from sudden cardiac arrest
The American Heart Association journal, Circulation, reported in November 2014 that in the United States, out-of-hospital cardiac arrest (OHCA) creates a huge burden on public health. Many of the victims are still in their productive years with approximately 350,000 OHCA deaths occurring each year and similar numbers in Europe. The impact of the financial burden on society is estimated at US$33 billion per year in the United States alone.

Apart from the costs of emergency response systems, for those who survive to reach hospital, there is a significant drain on resources with the additional costs of critical and intensive care, diagnostic tests and investigations and hospitalisation. For victims, who survive to be discharged from hospital, there are the costs of long-term care including rehabilitation, medical devices such as implantable cardioverter-defibrillators, disability expenses, and ongoing medical management.

If an employee dies from a cardiac arrest, the business will face potentially avoidable costs:

- to replace them
- to train their replacement
- in lost productivity, during the time the position is vacant.

Not all victims of SCA die – some will recover but the length of recovery time and the extent to which they resume normal life activities is directly affected by how long it takes for defibrillation to take place. Therefore, what might it cost if a staff member suffers cardiac arrest and is off sick, or can only return to limited duties, or is unable to return to work at all?

In December 2014, Ambulance Victoria released the *Victorian Ambulance Cardiac Arrest Registry annual report 2013–2014*. In a follow-up of survivors to assess their quality of life 12 months after a cardiac arrest, VACAR reported that 84% of those who survived to be discharged from hospital – after being defibrillated and revived within minutes of collapse by bystanders – returned to a normal productive life. In comparison, without early defibrillation less than 5% of victims even survive cardiac arrest, let alone return to normal life and activities. The value proposition of the investment in community participation in resuscitation is a very strong and powerful reason to have AEDs widely available. Together, we can make a difference.

A push for legislative change

Workplaces that have 10 or more employees (the minimum varies around Australia) are legally required to have first aid–trained officers. Therefore, if employers are required by law to train their staff to be competent in the use of AEDs, there is an inherent obligation upon them to also provide the equipment, so the first aid officers can perform their duties effectively and successfully.

In the 2012 *Joint statement on early access to defibrillation* (EAD) issued by the Australian Resuscitation Council, the National Heart Foundation of Australia and St John Ambulance Australia, the Australian, state and territory governments were called upon to support EAD by:

- Increas[ing] the number of AEDs that are accessible in places where large amounts of people frequent, such as train stations, casinos, sporting arenas, shopping centres, fitness centres, schools etc. and develop[ing] corresponding first responder programs that support their use
- Develop[ing] appropriate performance monitoring and feedback mechanisms which evaluate the ongoing effectiveness of EAD first responder programs
- Build[ing] community confidence in the use of AEDs through the implementation of community awareness campaigns that highlight both the misconceptions and benefits of prompt AED use
- Mandat[ing] the registration of all private and publically accessible AEDs, at the time of purchase, with local emergency service providers
- Develop[ing] a minimum standard to regulate the deployment of AEDs within large workplaces (over 200 employees) and to train employees in both AED use and CPR. (Appendix A)

As a nurse immuniser, I work in a wide variety of workplaces and corporate environments of varying size and staff numbers. Depending on the scale of the company, designated members of staff are appointed and trained as first aid officers who have a duty of care to respond to a first aid incident, especially an emergency situation. Some workplaces have voluntarily installed an AED; however, most have not.

According to the Australian Bureau of Statistics (ABS), 11.6 million people in Australia are in employment, and the majority of the population, both employed and unemployed, use retail, government, health, educational and sporting services. In other words, whether it is your own place of work or someone else's, you are accessing transport services, public spaces and workplaces every single day. Chapter 4 'Industry adoption of AEDs' looks at changing workplace attitudes to AEDs and highlights workplaces and public places where AEDs have saved lives.

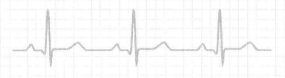

INDUSTRY ADOPTION OF AEDS

'Do something wonderful. People may imitate it.'

ALBERT SCHWEITZER

Despite a slow rate of deployment, support for lifesaving AEDs is gaining momentum across Australia and, particularly, the rest of the world.

Overseas, some state and local governments now require the placement of AEDs in public places such as shopping centres, transportation centres, entertainment precincts, and health and sports facilities. Airports have AEDs as standard first aid equipment. In Australia, AEDs are located in all sections of the airports including every transit lounge.

ANECDOTE: Urban Lifesavers take control at Melbourne Airport

At the Australian Resuscitation Council 2015 Spark of Life Conference in Melbourne, a very interesting and reassuring fact was revealed. For every cardiac arrest that has occurred at Melbourne Airport, it has been bystanders who have grabbed the AED from the wall and applied it to the victim before the airport response teams arrived. How remarkable is that? We can all be urban lifesaver heroes if we just know how simple it is to save a life.

Some jurisdictions have even passed laws protecting AED owners and people who use AEDs in an emergency. With growing awareness, the risk of potential liability resulting from not having an AED is becoming more likely.

In 2015, a lawsuit has been launched by a Hollywood executive's family alleging the gym where he died following a cardiac arrest was negligent for not having an AED available nor trained personnel. Since 2007, California law has required that the state's health clubs have an AED on site and maintained, as well as personnel trained in its use.[20]

Safe Work Australia is an Australian Government statutory agency established in 2009 as a national policy body (not a regulator of work health and safety). Safe Work Australia consists of representatives of the Australian, state and territory governments, the Australian Council of Trade Unions (ACTU), the Australian Chamber of Commerce and Industry and the Australian Industry Group. Safe Work Australia works with the Australian, state and territory governments to improve work health and safety and arrangements for workers' compensation.

In the March 2015 document *First aid in the workplace: code of practice*, Safe Work Australia noted that providing an AED can reduce the risk of fatality from cardiac arrest and is a useful addition for workplaces where there is a risk of electrocution or where there are large numbers of members of the public. It also noted that AEDs are designed to be used by trained or untrained persons.[21]

In the 2012 *Joint statement on early access to defibrillation*, it was noted that:

> In Australia, as with other countries around the world, first responder programs aimed at reducing the time to defibrillation have been successfully implemented ... These programs are linked with local emergency services to ensure the time to expert care is minimised. The first responder program implemented at the Melbourne Cricket Ground (MCG) [and the Shrine of Remembrance] is an excellent example of an effective systems approach to early defibrillation. This strategy has shown an 86% survival rate for cardiac arrest from first response to ambulance handover. (Appendix A)

There have been excellent outcomes around the world , such as King County, Seattle in the United States, when system-based policies have been implemented to minimise delays in access to advanced medical care in time-critical emergencies. These strategies are most successful when there is seamless government supported integration and collaboration between emergency and clinical heath care services.

The joint statement urged Australian, state and territory governments to support early access to defibrillation and improve survival rates by recommending the adoption of similar system-based approaches. To read the full *Joint statement on early access to defibrillation*, see Appendix A.

An example of changing attitudes – the Australian fitness industry

Fitness Australia is the national not-for-profit health and fitness industry association for registered businesses and exercise professionals. Fitness Australia governs and administers the National Exercise Professional Registration Scheme, Business Registration Scheme and Continuing Education Scheme, which are designed to safeguard the health and interests of people using fitness services. Fitness Australia's key functions are to provide a system of regulation for exercise professionals, businesses and education providers to ensure that they adhere to fitness industry standards and to promote best practice in the Australian fitness industry.

Fitness Australia's mission is to lead and represent the fitness industry in pursuit of a fitter, healthier nation and a better quality of life. Fitness Australia strives to support the fitness industry to deliver this commitment by being recognised for a high standard of customer care, safety and service as well as professionalism of the workforce and the quality of fitness facilities and businesses.[22]

Risk management

In the 2014 *Australian fitness industry risk management manual*, Fitness Australia recommends that being prepared for medical emergencies is crucial in reducing risk and potential liability. Fitness businesses and professionals have a professional and legal obligation to plan for and provide appropriate emergency care when these situations occur.[23]

Clear and effective communication between all personnel is essential for mitigating risk. Medical emergency action plans (EAPs) must be well documented and structured to foresee risks and guide first aid responders to identify and manage emergencies. No physical activity can be completely risk free, so it is important to develop and regularly review an EAP that is appropriate for the programs run by fitness facilities. The absence of an EAP, or an EAP that is not properly followed, could mean the difference between life and death for an individual. There may also be a basis for negligence claims.

A client suffering a cardiac arrest while exercising is one example of a potentially life-threatening injury that can occur without warning. Although rare, there is compelling 'evidence to indicate that vigorous physical activity acutely increases the risk of cardiovascular events among young individuals and adults with both occult (no symptoms) and diagnosed heart disease'.[24] Consequently, health and fitness centres are increasingly recognised as higher-risk sites that may benefit from placement of AEDs.

Fitness Australia recognises that AEDs used in the first few minutes of individuals suffering a SCA have been found to increase survival rates. While there are no laws in Australia requiring fitness centres to provide AEDs, it is recommended that fitness facilities should at least consider installing and using AEDs. Several international and professional organisations have 'strongly encouraged' larger centres to install them, which is particularly important if the clientele are older or have a 'high-risk' profile, for example, clients with cardiovascular, respiratory or metabolic disease. International negligence case law and duty of care principles suggest the standard of care required in health/fitness centres may be increasing.

> Research suggests that it is crucial that the staff also receive re-training and refresher courses obtained from accredited education providers in order to ensure the retention and knowledge in skills required to use AEDs. It is also advised that the AEDs should be well maintained in accordance with the manufacturers' recommendations, local laws and regulations.[25]

Responsible and responsive workplaces

A tragic workplace death in 2012 prompted a South Australian coroner to call upon employers to ensure that all staff members know where to find an AED (if available) and also have appropriate training in how to use it. In this instance, a man collapsed in cardiac arrest and his colleagues, who had first aid training, attempted to revive him with CPR. They did not, however, use the AED that was on a wall in an office and defibrillation was not attempted until paramedics arrived, at which time it was too late.

The coroner, Mark Johns, stated, 'I wish to draw this matter to the attention of the general public, to ensure that where defibrillators are available to be used as a possible means of resuscitation, their actual use should be encouraged'.[26]

BASF Australia
BASF Australia is an example of a responsible and responsive employer. In 2013, BASF's Cheltenham site purchased an AED when it was identified during a first aid training session that the location of the nearest unit was a considerable distance away.

After the AED was installed, BASF staff informed neighbouring companies that BASF had purchased an AED and that it was available to them in case of an emergency.

Only weeks later, a client at the gym right next door suffered a SCA. The AED was retrieved and the client was defibrillated before emergency medical services (EMS) arrived. The story of BASF's commitment to safety and details of the citations awarded to staff members from BASF and the gym are covered in Chapter 19 'Myth 7 – An AED in the workplace increases liability'.

CASE STUDY: Samantha Jobe

The case of 32-year-old new mother Samantha (Sam) Jobe clearly demonstrates the effectiveness of having an emergency action plan and applying early defibrillation. On 10 May 2014, Sam attended the Crossfit121 fitness centre at Cheltenham, Melbourne, accompanied by her husband, Damien, and two-month-old baby daughter, Makayla. Sam had just started her ropes workout when she suffered a sudden cardiac arrest and collapsed to the floor. The trainers of the gym, Maria, Chris and Tara immediately called Triple Zero (000) and started cardiopulmonary resuscitation (CPR).

The gym did not have an AED but, fortunately for everyone, the business next door, BASF, had purchased an AED only weeks earlier when they identified that the location of the nearest AED unit was a considerable distance away. BASF had then informed all the local businesses where the AED was located. The AED was retrieved from BASF and used to defibrillate Sam. The first aid management of Sam's cardiac arrest was textbook perfect.

Sam survived and now has an implanted defibrillator which has saved her life a second time when it detected a lethal heart rhythm and automatically defibrillated her early enough to prevent her suffering another full cardiac arrest. It is important to note that Sam did not have a heart attack; the cause of her cardiac arrest is believed to be an abnormal heart rhythm or electrical disturbance of her heartbeat. Cardiac arrests in younger people are rarely caused by a heart attack and if defibrillated quickly a young person's abnormal heart rhythm can be effectively reversed. Too many young victims do not survive, however, because AEDs are not available quickly enough.

Chris and Maria have since purchased an AED for their Crossfit121 centre and I have provided additional training for their staff.

Asda stores, United Kingdom

In a 2014 groundbreaking partnership with the British Heart Foundation (BHF), Asda became the first retailer to roll out defibrillators into all of their 609 stores, warehouses and offices across the United Kingdom, giving their employees and 18 million customers the best chance of survival if cardiac arrest strikes.[27]

A public access defibrillator (PAD) or AED can be used by any member of the public to deliver a lifesaving electric shock to someone's heart when they've suffered a cardiac arrest. BHF Chief Executive, Simon Gillespie, said:

Cardiac arrest survival rates in the UK are astonishingly low. But Asda's bold commitment to become the first large retailer to have CPR trained staff and public access defibrillators in every store will be instrumental in helping communities up and down the country access the life-saving support they need in an emergency. This really could mean the difference between life and death for someone having a cardiac arrest while doing something as ordinary as shopping.[28]

AEDs are exceptionally easy to use, enabling people of all ages and walks of life to provide emergency care to victims of cardiac arrest, quickly and effectively, before an ambulance arrives. There is a problem, however,' as nearly three-quarters of the population are not trained in CPR [cardiopulmonary resuscitation] and the evidence indicates that 'public access defibrillators are available in just 4% of cardiac arrests'. The BHF believes 'far more needs to be done to give people a better chance of survival … [and] will work with local ambulance trusts to run familiarisation training for 12,000 Asda colleagues on how to use an AED as part of the full chain of survival'. [29]

Over 60,000 cardiac arrests occur outside of hospital every year in the United Kingdom with only ten percent of victims surviving. Research has shown that potentially 75%–85% of people who suffer cardiac arrests can be revived by defibrillation if the chain of survival is followed quickly with an immediate call to emergency services, early CPR, early defibrillation and proper post-resuscitation care.

The more quickly a victim of cardiac arrest is defibrillated, not only is their chance of survival improved but also their likelihood of making a full recovery. For every minute a victim is in cardiac arrest, the chance of survival decreases by 9%–10% so it is important that people don't just know where AEDs are located but also know how to use them. The move to locate AEDs in Asda stores, warehouses and offices will reduce the amount of time shoppers, staff members and people in surrounding communities have to wait for these lifesaving interventions if a cardiac arrest strikes in or around an Asda store.[30]

At Asda Tunstall, England, the AED has already been used to save a staff member who suffered a cardiac arrest in store and has made a full recovery.[31] Another two lives have been saved at Asda stores by members of the public and Asda staff in April and May 2015.

Asda are clear on their community objectives. Their stores need to:

- be responsible to community
- promote safety
- save a life if they can by providing and knowing how to use the AED.

Bendigo Bank Community Enterprise Foundation
Another organisation that has embraced corporate social responsibility, with a commitment to the amateur sporting community, is the Community Enterprise Foundation branch of the Bendigo Bank in Australia. The foundation has contributed large sums of money to support community sporting clubs through the not-for-profit organisation Defib Your Club, For Life! Sports groups have been able to obtain grants through the Bendigo Bank to purchase an AED for their club which has greatly increased the number of AEDs available in sporting facilities throughout the country.

Development of a minimum standard governing AED uptake within the workplace

In 2000, United States President Bill Clinton signed the Federal Cardiac Arrest Survival Act 2000 (US) which requires AEDs to be placed in all federal facilities.[32] Fifteen years later, no minimum standard for AEDs within the workplace (including government sites) currently exists within Australia. However, the 2012 *Joint statement on early access to defibrillation* recommended that to foster the uptake of AEDs within the workplace, a minimum standard should be developed which clearly outlines AEDs as a key component of workplace occupational health and safety (see Appendix A). According to the joint statement, a minimum standard governing larger workplaces (minimum 200 employees), could encompass the following areas, similar to the regulation of fire extinguishers:

- accessibility (i.e. location and height)
- visibility
- maintenance
- minimum number of staff trained in AED use.

The joint statement further stated that regular training of workplace staff in CPR and AED use was recommended as standard organisational best practice. Australian employers are encouraged to be proactive in the implementation of AEDs within their workplaces. The joint statement concluded that early access to defibrillation is vital to improving outcomes from SCA. AEDs in the public domain have been shown to save lives with first responder programs being effective in reducing time to defibrillation. Early intervention results in fewer complications and enables a smooth handover to paramedic emergency services with enhanced likelihood of successful hospital care.

Within Australia, AEDs are currently accessible in major airports, transport hubs, shopping centres, major sporting arenas and a growing list of community groups and sporting clubs. Similar to statements issued by the BHF, the joint statement also called for AEDs to be accessible in places considered high risk of a SCA, such as health and fitness centres. Regular exercise is beneficial for cardiac health; however, 'evidence suggests that heavy physical exertion in some people may be a "trigger" for an acute coronary event and subsequent cardiac arrest' (Appendix A).

In their 2012 joint statement, St John Ambulance Australia, the Australian Resuscitation Council and the National Heart Foundation of Australia called upon the Australian, state and territory governments to take the lead in developing and implementing early access defibrillation policy, to ensure that over 30,000 Australians who suffer out-of-hospital cardiac arrest (OHCA) every year are given the best chance of survival (see Appendix A).

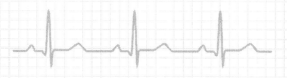

CHAPTER 5

SUMMARY OF WORKPLACE CONCERNS AND OBLIGATIONS

'Ask yourself what is really important and then have the wisdom and courage to build your life around your answer.'

LEE JAMPOLSKY

What are the concerns held by employers, their staff and customers about providing an AED in the workplace? What are the obligations and benefits for employers, their staff and customers? How does providing an AED in the workplace affect the risks?

A workplace has a duty of care to its employees, volunteers and visitors. Employers and government agencies are required to provide the safest working environment possible. But defibrillation must be provided within the first three to five minutes of a sudden cardiac arrest to give the greatest likelihood of success, so how can an organisation claim to be providing a safe environment when an AED isn't available, should it be needed? How does this meet an organisation's obligation to protect the safety of employees and customers, in particular in large organisations that have hundreds and even thousands of people attending their premises every day?

Damage can potentially be caused to the brand and reputation of an organisation should a cardiac arrest occur on their premises and the victim dies because the lifesaving equipment is not available. This is a particular concern to organisations with high public and media profiles that espouse values of caring for the community. To be identified as a concerned, safety-conscious organisation that does not provide lifesaving equipment could be detrimental to public confidence in their brand.

Workplaces are increasingly being identified as avenues for health promotion and health education for the workforce in Australia (Victoria's WorkHealth program is an example of this approach). First aid training and the availability of critical equipment should be integral to this philosophy.

With increased awareness of the changes to training regulations and the importance of early defibrillation, and as the availability of AEDs grows, the likelihood of a negligence lawsuit is increasing should a death result because lifesaving equipment was not provided on site. The costs could be far greater than the modest outlay to buy an AED and train staff in its use.

Following changes to first aid training regulations, it is inevitable that OH&S/WHS laws will be amended with respect to provision of AEDs, and workplaces need to consider the potential risks associated with safety, liability, governance and compliance if they don't have a defibrillator as part of the first aid kit.

AEDs save lives and provide a sustainable benefit to the community. They enhance and promote safety, reduce lost time injury, improve staff morale by instilling confidence that they are in a safe and responsible workplace, and promote a sense of family security in that workers are more likely to return home to their families. AEDs also protect the bottom line by providing practical insurance against lost productivity and the additional costs of sickness/termination payments and retraining new staff.

It is mandatory for workplaces to provide and maintain fire extinguishers in the workplace. As previously stated, when comparing 33,000 cardiac arrests each year with 56 deaths caused by fire or smoke,[33] individuals are 590 times more likely to suffer a sudden cardiac arrest than die in a fire so why would the workplace *not* provide an AED? Early defibrillation is the most vital yet the most frequently missing link in the chain of survival. There is a duty of care incumbent upon the employer to provide the equipment that first aid officers have been trained to use, but without an AED, first aid officers cannot provide the only effective treatment for a cardiac arrest.

AED technology has improved so dramatically in recent years that bystanders can safely and effectively use AEDs to save lives without waiting for paramedics to arrive. (Changes in technology are described in Chapter 9 'History of defibrillation to present day technology'.) Until the law catches up with the advancements in technology and minimum standards are established, it is up to individual workplaces to step up and install AEDs not just for their staff but also as a community service, similar to the initiatives undertaken by the Asda retail chain, BASF and the Bendigo Bank Community Enterprise Foundation.

More discussion on the issues affecting placement of AEDs in workplaces can be found in Chapter 19 'Myth 7 – An AED in the workplace increases liability'.

Part Two

SUDDEN CARDIAC ARREST

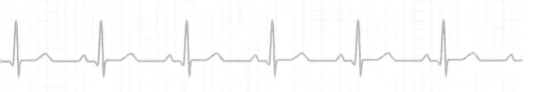

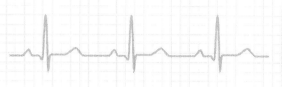

CHAPTER 6

WHAT IS SUDDEN CARDIAC ARREST?

*'And out of darkness came the hands that
reach thro' nature, moulding men.'*

ALFRED LORD TENNYSON

Facts and statistics

Sudden cardiac arrest (SCA):

- means the heart (cardiac) unexpectedly (sudden) stops (arrest)
- is a lethal abnormality in the electrical impulse which controls the pumping action of the heart
- is a separate event from a heart attack, although it can be caused by heart attack
- can occur at any age without prior warning signs or symptoms
- is reversible, but without treatment always results in *death*.

Early defibrillation is vital because:

- without early defibrillation, less than 5% of cardiac arrest victims will survive
- defibrillation within the first few minutes increases survival rate dramatically to 70%–85%.

Without effective pumping or circulation of blood, the person experiencing a SCA will suddenly collapse, lose consciousness, appear lifeless, stop breathing (exception: sometimes there can be abnormal 'gasping' which may last for a short time) and will have no pulse. Occasionally, victims of SCA will display 10–20 seconds of seizures or spasms ('fitting' – shaking or jerking of the body, arms and legs) at the onset of the event as the supply of blood and oxygen to the brain is depleted.

A victim of SCA is *never awake* and their condition rapidly progresses to irreversible heart and brain damage then death, if there is no immediate rescue intervention.

An introduction to your heart

The human heart is a muscle about the size of a clenched fist, which lies in the middle of the chest behind the breastbone (sternum), slightly to the left of centre. It is divided into four internal cavities or compartments, known as the cardiac chambers, which contain blood.

The heart (cardiac) muscle pumps the blood by contracting or squeezing the four chambers in a controlled, rhythmic and regular sequence. The circulation of blood is pumped in a closed system of blood vessels that transport blood around the body and return it to the heart under pressure, that is, blood pressure. The coordinated squeezing action of the heart muscle creates the blood pressure, which forces the blood out of the heart's chambers into the circulation (via the arteries) and allows the blood to return to the heart (via the veins). This cycle is maintained throughout a person's lifespan. The average person's heart circulates their entire volume of blood around the circulatory system – away from and back to the heart – every minute.

All muscles and organs need an adequate blood supply to bring them nutrients and oxygen so they can function effectively. The heart is no different – it is a muscle as well as a vital organ and must have a supply of oxygenated blood in order to stay healthy and keep functioning, so that it can pump the blood volume within its chambers out through the arteries around the body and back to the heart through the veins. That is how we stay alive.

Four chambers of the heart

The four chambers that collect the blood are divided into two upper and two lower compartments. The upper chambers are called the right atrium and left atrium (pronounced 'ay-tree-um'; plural *atria*, pron.

'ay-tree-ah'). The atria are the collecting 'reservoirs' or 'dams' of the heart. Reserve supplies of blood are constantly flowing back into the atria under pressure created by the heart's contractions. The atria contract together and empty blood into the two lower chambers, the right ventricle and left ventricle (pronounced 'ven-tri-kl'; plural *ventricles*). The ventricles are the powerhouses of the heart. They are responsible for contracting together, creating blood pressure and forcefully expelling blood from the heart out to the lungs or to the rest of the body, delivering effective blood circulation.

Two pumps in the heart

The heart is also divided into two sides, left and right, with an atrium and a ventricle on each side, creating two pumps which operate in unison. The right-side pump receives the oxygen-depleted blood returning from the rest of the body. When the right ventricle contracts, it pumps the blood it contains to the lungs where the blood is replenished with oxygen. The left-side pump receives the oxygenated blood back from the lungs and, when the left ventricle contracts, it pumps the newly oxygenated blood out to the body.

Electrical signals that control the heartbeat

How and when the heart muscle pumps is controlled by an electrical signal or impulse which emanates from a small node at the top of the heart, called the sino-atrial node (SA node). The SA node is the 'natural pacemaker' for the heart in that it determines the speed (pace) at which the heart contracts. This electrical impulse is generated autonomously and is not under the conscious control of the brain. We can choose to hold our breath and stop breathing for a period; however, we cannot turn the SA node off or on at will. It is out of our control and operates throughout our entire lives.

The heart muscle is made up of millions of cardiac cells which respond in a coordinated sequence to the electrical signal as it travels down pathways through the heart muscle. The SA node releases the electrical impulse at the top of the heart and first stimulates the two upper chambers (the atria) to contract and push their volume of blood into the two lower chambers (the ventricles). The electrical impulses then relay down conduction pathways within the heart muscle and stimulate the muscle of the ventricles to contract and pump blood out of the heart. This cycle creates a regular heart rhythm and blood pressure which pushes or circulates blood around the body. Each time the heart muscle contracts as a result of a stimulus from the SA node, a pulse can be felt at various points in the body.

As the electrical stimulus fades away from the chambers of the heart between heartbeats, there is a moment of rest for the heart's chambers to relax and refill with blood (called 'cardiac refill') in time for the next electrical impulse which causes the next heartbeat. In a normally functioning heart, this process repeats itself from the earliest weeks of pregnancy throughout the person's lifespan until they die. The SA node increases its rate in response to stimuli such as exercise, agitation/ excitement, stimulant drugs or fever, and decreases its rate when the body is at rest or asleep.

What does a normal heart rhythm look like?
In the diagram, the tracing represents an electrocardiogram (ECG) recording of a normal heart rhythm known as sinus rhythm (*electro* = electrical activity; *cardio* = heart; *gram* = recording). Each complex or spike (QRS) occurs when the SA node emits its electrical impulse to cause the heart to contract or beat. In other words, each (QRS) spike represents the ventricles contracting and can be felt as a pulse. ('P' is the electrical activity of the atria contracting and 'T' is the recovery of the ventricles ready for the next contraction.)

The distance between two spikes (QRS) is the cardiac refill (time interval between contractions) during which the chambers of the heart refill with blood ready for the next contraction.

Every pulse we feel results from a heartbeat and represents the electrical stimulus that has caused that heartbeat.

(Although it will be covered in more detail later, it is important to note that if an AED was applied to anyone and it detected a normal heart rhythm, the device *would not* advise *or* deliver a shock.)

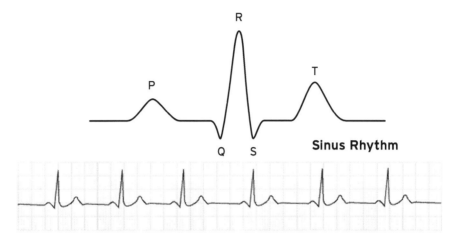

Figure 2. ECG showing normal heart rhythm

What happens to the heart rhythm during a sudden cardiac arrest?
Transmission problems with the electrical signal in the heart muscle can be caused by disease, trauma or abnormalities of the electrical conducting system, and can occur at any point along the heart's conduction pathway. Abnormally conducted signals are irregular, aberrant rhythms known medically as *arrhythmias* (pronounced 'ay-rith-mee-uhz') and they alter the heart's normal beating action, which can be seen on the ECG recordings.

SCA is triggered by a malfunction of the electrical system which causes the heart muscle to quiver or 'fibrillate' instead of pump normally. A victim of cardiac arrest is clinically dead.

SCA occurs when the electrical impulse that stimulates the heart to contract in a regular rhythm becomes disrupted. This causes the millions of heart muscles cells to behave erratically and start firing off chaotic electrical energy without any coordination, pattern or sequence. SCA is fatal because the heartbeat abruptly stops, the blood pressure drops to zero and the heart's chambers are no longer being refilled with blood. The heart muscle is no longer contracting so it cannot squeeze the blood out into circulation around the body, especially to the vital organs such as the brain and heart.

Ventricular tachycardia

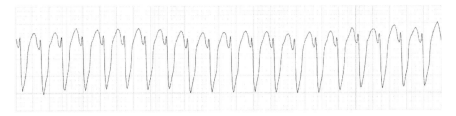

Figure 3. ECG showing ventricular tachycardia
(Image reproduced with kind permission of Vince Di Giulio)

In Figure 3, the rapid electrical impulses are causing the heart's ventricles to contract too quickly. This is known as ventricular tachycardia (VT) (from Latin – *tach*y = fast; *cardia* = heart). Although the heart rhythm still has a regular pattern of spikes representing contractions of the heart muscle, the contractions are so fast that there is not enough time between beats for the chambers of the heart to refill with a sufficient volume of blood. As a result, each fast contraction expels less blood than the contraction before. The heartbeat then gets faster and faster to try to compensate for the lack of blood volume and flow.

The heart cannot continue to beat at this rate because the muscle cells become more irritable due to the lack of blood supply and oxygen. VT will rapidly progress to ventricular fibrillation (VF), which is fatal.

Ventricular fibrillation

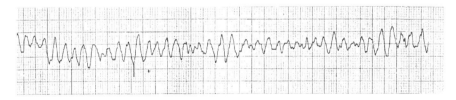

Figure 4. ECG showing ventricular fibrillation
(Image reproduced with kind permission of Vince Di Giulio)

Ventricular fibrillation (VF) occurs when the electrical signals within the heart suddenly become completely chaotic and control of the pumping function is lost. VF is rapid, uncontrolled electrical activity/contraction of individual muscle cells with little or no movement of the heart muscle as a whole. There is, therefore, no effective pumping of blood to the brain, lungs and other organs.

Although VF is instantaneous death, it is reversible because both VT and VF are shockable rhythms. In other words, an AED would detect and recognise the abnormal rhythms VT and VF, and would deliver a shock to reinstate the normal heart rhythm.

Restoring electrical activity to normal

The most critically important point is that the heart muscle cells are still electrically active – there is still a tracing on the ECG and not a flat-line which would indicate no electrical activity. Although electrical energy is still present in the heart, it is in a dysfunctional, quivering state that does not allow the heart to contract effectively to pump and circulate blood. A quick combination of CPR and defibrillation can, in most cases, restore life.

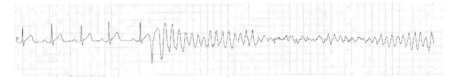

Figure 5. An example of a normal heart rhythm suddenly
going into ventricular tachycardia (VT) and rapidly progressing to
ventricular fibrillation (VF), that is, cardiac arrest
(Image reproduced with kind permission of Vince Di Giulio)

Ventricular fibrillation vs. atrial fibrillation

When we refer to ventricular fibrillation (VF), the term 'ventricular' is derived from the name of the lower heart chambers, which are responsible for pumping blood out of the heart.

The less serious condition of atrial fibrillation (AF) is derived from the name of the upper heart chambers (the atria), so the term AF refers to the atria (not the ventricles) fibrillating.

AF and VF are not the same condition. Although both need to be medically treated, the heart can be in AF with the ventricles pumping normally. VF, however, is instantaneously fatal.

Risk factors for sudden cardiac arrest

SCA can strike anyone, of any age, anytime, anywhere. In the United States of America, SCA is associated with the following risk factors, which can be extrapolated to similar industrialised societies:

- Out-of-hospital cardiac arrest (OHCA) occurrence per 10,000 adults is 10.1 among African Americans, 6.5 among Hispanic people and 5.8 among Caucasian people.
- Pre-existing cardiac disease poses a significant risk factor for cardiac arrest.
- Potential risk of cardiac arrest is double if there is a family history of cardiac arrest, in a first-degree relative (parents, offspring, siblings).[34]

What causes sudden cardiac arrest?

During the normal expected end stages of life (that is, when it is known that death is imminent) death occurs when the heart ceases to beat. All deaths end in cardiac arrest. Sudden cardiac arrest, however, is an unexpected event with many causes. SCA is defined as the unexpected cessation of cardiac mechanical activity, in other words, the pumping or contraction of the heart muscle stops. SCA is confirmed by the absence of signs of circulation – the victim has no breathing or pulse. Traditionally, the causes of SCA fall into two categories: cardiac or non-cardiac origin.

A SCA is presumed to be of cardiac origin – caused by a problem with the heart itself – unless it is known or likely that the SCA was caused by trauma, submersion (drowning), inhalation of smoke or fumes, drug overdose, asphyxia, severe blood loss, or any other non-cardiac cause.[35]

Cardiac arrest can result from:

- genetic disorders
- cardiac arrhythmias (abnormal heartbeats)
- stroke
- heart attack/coronary artery disease
- asphyxiation from fumes or smoke
- electrocution
- drowning

- asthma attack
- severe bleeding or fluid loss causing shock
- choking/strangulation
- drug overdose/poisoning
- anaphylaxis
- injury, such as a car accident
- unknown causes
- suffocation or any circumstance that causes a person to stop breathing.

Three examples of causes of SCA are:

Long QT syndrome

Long QT syndrome (LQTS) is a genetic disorder of the heart's electrical activity. LQTS is a common underlying, undiagnosed heart rhythm abnormality which can sometimes be triggered by exercise and stress. It can cause a sudden, uncontrollable, dangerous arrhythmia that results from an interval in the heartbeat being longer than normal, which can then upset the careful timing of the heartbeat and trigger the dangerous heart rhythms. Not everyone who has LQTS has dangerous heart rhythms but when they do occur, they can be fatal. Implanted defibrillators are often used to control LQTS.[36]

Hypertrophic cardiomyopathy

Hypertrophic cardiomyopathy (HCM) is a congenital heart muscle disease. The walls of the heart's left ventricle become abnormally thickened (hypertrophy). The structural abnormality can lead to obstruction of blood flow from the heart, causing loss of consciousness and irregular heartbeat, leading to SCA.

HCM caused the death of our long-time close friend Karen Rizzoli, who was 53 years old when she suffered a cardiac arrest in her sleep on 5 January 2008. It was our daughter's birthday and just six weeks later we would be struck again with the sudden death of my husband, Paul, whose cardiac arrest was caused by a heart attack.

HCM also affects two of Karen's three daughters, Janelle and Angela, who both have implanted defibrillators as a precaution.

Commotio cordis – traumatic cause

Commotio cordis is Latin for 'agitation of the heart'. A fatal disruption of heart rhythm follows an impact to the chest above the heart, at a specific and critical time during the cycle of a heartbeat, causing cardiac arrest. It is a form of ventricular fibrillation (VF) and is not the result of heart disease. It affects mostly boys and young men, usually during sports (most often baseball in the United States).

Commotio cordis most commonly results from the impact with a projectile such as a cricket ball, baseball or football and even from the blow of an elbow or other body part. Even if the victim is wearing chest protection equipment, they may still not be safe. The rib cage of an adolescent is more prone to this type of injury because their chests are less developed.[37]

The fatality rate for commotio cordis is about 65% but it can often be reversed by early defibrillation. At the US Commotio Cordis Registry, researchers studied 124 cases and found the average age of victims was 14 with only 18 survivors (14%), most of whom had received prompt CPR and defibrillation.[38]

In recent years, two incidents of commotio cordis in Melbourne, Australia, had very different outcomes.

CASE STUDIES: Commotio cordis in young people

In August 2011, a 17-year-old Bacchus Marsh (Victoria) player suffered a cardiac arrest during a football game after a bump to the chest. It took 20 minutes for paramedics to reach the player with a defibrillator and he couldn't be revived.

In March 2012, a 25-year-old cricketer was struck in the chest during cricket training in Greensborough (Melbourne). This story was another one of mixed luck. He was unlucky to be hit by a speeding cricket ball, and even more unlucky to be struck in the chest. In another stroke of bad luck, he took the hit just over his heart. The final bit of bad luck was that the ball hit him at the precise moment of his heartbeat that can result in a cardiac arrest. Luckily, although it was more than 10 minutes before paramedics arrived, they were able to revive the young man with a defibrillator.

How can sudden cardiac arrest be prevented?

Living a healthy lifestyle – exercising regularly, eating healthy foods, maintaining a reasonable weight, and avoiding smoking – can help prevent cardiovascular disease (CVD). Monitoring and controlling blood pressure, cholesterol levels and diabetes is also important. It is important to not ignore family history and potential inherited disorders. If a pre-disposition for cardiac conditions exists, it is advisable to seek specialist assessment and management of the risks.

If abnormal heart rhythms or arrhythmias are detected, they can be treated through implantable cardioverter-defibrillator (ICD) therapy, use of medications, and surgical intervention, for example catheter ablation which is a procedure to remove the abnormal electrical activity and permit the victim to live a normal life.[39]

Can victims of sudden cardiac arrest recover to live a normal life?

SCA is a critical public health issue and, fortunately, it is reversible most of the time with immediate CPR and prompt use of an AED to jolt the victim back to life. Bystanders need to act quickly because after the victim has been in cardiac arrest for approximately four to six minutes, irreversible brain and tissue damage may begin to occur. For every minute a person is in cardiac arrest without being successfully defibrillated, their chance of survival decreases by 9%–10%.

Response times for most ambulances in Australia are on average greater than 10 minutes, so an ambulance may not arrive during the critical few minutes in which the casualty's life can be saved. The delay in arrival of paramedics does not mean that the victim cannot survive with only CPR and without early defibrillation, but the chances of survival are drastically reduced the longer the time progresses. An AED is most effective if applied within three to five minutes of collapse.

Even the fastest emergency medical services may not be able to reach a victim this quickly, which is why prompt action by bystanders is so critical and why it is so important that more laypersons learn CPR and how to use an AED.

In Denmark following an increase in public access AEDs from 141 in 2007 to 7,800 in 2012 along with improved education and awareness of CPR, survival of cardiac arrest victims, following bystander use of an AED, has risen from less than 10% in 2001 to around 55% in 2012.[40]

Studies in Japan and North Carolina, United States support the findings that an increase in bystander CPR directly affects survival and improved neurological outcomes.

King County, Seattle in the United States reported a 62% survival rate in 2013 from cardiac arrest due in part to increased bystander CPR and early defibrillation with public access AEDs.

In the long-term functional outcomes reported by the Victorian Ambulance Cardiac Arrest Registry (VACAR), 84% of adult out-of-hospital cardiac arrest (OHCA) cases who were known to survive and be transported to hospital were discharged home. In 2014, follow-up phone interviews showed that the majority of survivors maintained their independence and had a good quality of life 12 months after their cardiac arrest. Most people who survive SCA can return to their previous level of functioning. All survivors need follow-up care with physicians who specialise in heart conditions (cardiologists and electrophysiologists).

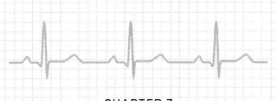

CHAPTER 7

SUDDEN CARDIAC ARREST IN YOUNG PEOPLE

'First say to yourself what you would be;
and then do what you have to do.'

EPICTETUS

It is less well known to the general public that SCA also affects young people who have underlying and unrecognised genetic abnormalities of the electrical system that controls the heart's function. Many people have pre-existing medical conditions or known heart disease that place them at risk of suffering a SCA. It can also occur in the one in 7,000 young and active people who seem to be healthy and have no known medical conditions. In these younger people, SCA is the first indication of a cardiac problem.

Sudden arrhythmic death syndrome

Sudden arrhythmic death syndrome (SADS) occurs in people usually aged between 12 and 35 years. Elite athletes with abnormal hearts are particularly vulnerable, especially during physical exertion. When these deaths do occur, it is often while participating in a sporting event or competition involving physical activity. There have been multiple deaths around the world of fit, young athletes taking part in marathons and triathlons. It is not the sport or stress that causes the cardiac arrest but rather the individual's previously unknown underlying cardiac condition which can be triggered by physical exertion or emotional stress and can result in the life-threatening abnormal heart rhythm.

Importance of early defibrillation

Numerous amateur footballers and club members have died in Australia in recent years after suffering sudden cardiac arrest and not having immediate access to defibrillation.

CASE STUDY: Stephen Buckman

Tragic loss of Stephen Buckman led to the establishment of Defib For Life!

In May 2010, 19-year-old Stephen Buckman felt unwell and came off the ground during football training at his local amateur club in Rupertswood, Victoria. He collapsed in sudden cardiac arrest in the clubrooms. Off-duty mobile intensive care ambulance (MICA) paramedic Andrew White (who was also a parent/member of the club) and a doctor performed CPR for 22 minutes until an ambulance arrived with a defibrillator.

Although the CPR was effective and maintained good colour and blood circulation (perfusion), it was unfortunately too late to revert Stephen's heart to a normal rhythm. Stephen was a fit and healthy young man and the first anyone knew that he had an underlying cardiac arrhythmia disorder was when he died. Stephen's younger sister, Ashlea, now has an implanted defibrillator after being diagnosed with the same cardiac disorder.

Defib Your Club, For Life! is a not-for-profit organisation that was established that year in Stephen's memory by Andrew White and Stephen's mother, Sue Buckman, to raise awareness about sudden cardiac arrest, distribute AEDs to sporting and voluntary clubs, and promote a public access defibrillation program.

As a first aid trainer, I am very proud to be associated with Defib Your Club, For Life!, recently re-branded as Defib For Life, by delivering AED information sessions for organisations that install defibrillators on their premises.

The following case studies are typical examples of previously healthy young people who suddenly died due to undiagnosed heart conditions and who were saved by early defibrillation.

A Melbourne high school student went into cardiac arrest and fell into a lake during a cross-country running event in September 2011. The student is one of the rare lucky cases: he was kept alive with CPR for about 10 minutes by two teachers until paramedics arrived with a defibrillator. He survived and is now fitted with an implanted defibrillator.

On 5 March 2012, a young woman in her mid-twenties was walking along Chapel Street, one of Melbourne's busiest shopping strips, around 8:30 pm, when she suddenly collapsed in cardiac arrest. A group of shoppers including a doctor started CPR. The doctor retrieved an AED from a nearby shopping centre and used it to shock and revive the young woman.

Another young victim of sudden cardiac arrest (in his early 20s) was at home in Melbourne in December 2013 and luckily, his teenage younger brother happened to be ill and home from school that day. The teenager heard a loud thud and found his older brother unconscious and unresponsive on the floor. He called Triple Zero (000) and with advice from the emergency medical services (EMS) operator, he performed CPR on his brother. Fortunately an ambulance arrived within eight minutes and paramedics were able to defibrillate the victim and revive him.

Following five reported deaths on New South Wales sporting fields in 2014 and almost as many up till September in 2015, the National Rugby League (NRL) and the Australian Football League (AFL), supported by cricket and netball groups, have jointly called on the NSW State Government to provide AEDs to all sporting grounds. NSW ambulance data shows that 76 cardiac arrests occurred on a sports field in 2012, which is more than one a week. Following a report that, eight males had died on NSW sporting fields between February 2014 – May 2015, *The Sunday Telegraph* newspaper launched on online petition on www.change.org to gather support for the rollout of AEDs into all NSW sporting clubs.[41]

There have also been multiple sporting related deaths following cardiac arrest in Victoria in recent months (2015) and the Victorian State Government has committed to supplying 1000 AEDs to sports clubs starting in 2016. Rolling out defibrillators will not, however, be enough.

Support for AEDs at sporting venues

A statement issued in February 2011 by Dr David O'Donnell MBBS, FRACP, FCSANZ, cardiologist and electrophysiologist at the Department of Cardiology, Austin Hospital, Melbourne, supported the distribution of AEDs in the community. Dr O'Donnell views remain current in 2015. He wrote:

> Sudden cardiac death is the number one killer in most developed countries including Australia. As a Cardiologist and Electrophysiologist, I spend my professional career trying to identify and treat patients at high risk of sudden cardiac death and to manage the lucky few who actually survive a potentially fatal cardiac arrest. In addition I work closely with a number of sporting bodies and sporting teams to reduce the risk of sudden cardiac death.

> Clearly exercise is beneficial to many aspects of life. It is recognized, however, that at peaks of exertion the heart is put under stress and in certain individuals this can lead to cardiac arrest. Without access to automatic external defibrillators, the vast majority of these individuals will not survive. Those who do survive can be treated and expect to live a close to normal and productive life.

> The vast majority of patients who experience sudden cardiac events die before reaching medical attention. It has repeatedly been shown that one of the best predictors of survival is time to successful defibrillation. This has led to the utilization of Automatic External Defibrillators (AEDs) at airports, major sporting venues, the offices of many large corporations and the private homes of interested individuals. It is a little incongruous that all of these areas have AEDs but we are exposing our young athletes to risk without any protection.

> AEDs distributed across the Victorian community and at sporting venues will save lives.

> The cost effectiveness of this strategy will compare favourably with many medical interventions and prove much more cost effective than most present screening strategies.

> I am fully supportive of the principle to utilize AEDs across the Victorian community and would be happy to provide detailed scientific information to support this initiative if requested.

Education and training are critical to ensure that as many people as possible are confident and knowledgeable in the use of AEDs.

Tasmanian emergency services have joined forces to coordinate access to early defibrillation, with over 500 AEDs now registered in the state, representing one AED per 1,000 people. The objective is to provide the best cardiac arrest response times in the world.[42]

Incidence of heart abnormalities

It is estimated that one in 1000 people of all ages will have an undiagnosed cardiac abnormality. That is not to say that one in every 1000 will have a SCA, but for some of those individuals the first indication that they do have an underlying cardiac condition is when they suffer a cardiac arrest. It is possible, however, for some people to be screened and identified in advance as being at risk for SCA.

Survival rates among young people

In the United States, there are an estimated 7,000 cardiac arrest fatalities in children each year. Among young people (<18 years old) who have a cardiac arrest, only 5.4% survive to hospital discharge. The majority of cardiac arrests in young people are caused by a heart rhythm malfunction which is reversible if treated quickly with defibrillation. The 5.4% survival rate could dramatically improve to over 80% if rapid defibrillation with an AED was available at the scene. Without early defibrillation, the victim's chances of survival diminish during delays waiting for EMS to arrive.

AEDs in schools

In 2007, following the deaths of four children in two months in 2006 with a total of 15 children dying in the whole year, the state of Texas in the United States passed the most comprehensive AED bill (SB82) in the country, requiring every private, elementary, middle and high school in the state to have a defibrillator and staff members to know where to find it and are trained to use it. The Bill also stipulates that AEDs be readily accessible and not locked away. It took for the sixteenth child to finally be saved by an AED for action to be taken.[43]

Managing the risk of SADS with preventative measures

In a February 2012 media report following the death of a young footballer caused by Commotio Cordis, the Australian Resuscitation Council's Professor Peter Morley stated that 'cardiac arrest can happen to anyone, at any time but [for young people] was more likely to occur during vigorous physical exercise in competitive sports such as football, basketball and athletics. [Cycling is another high-risk activity] ... 'Having a defibrillator on site is critical in giving players suffering a cardiac arrest the best possible chance of survival and recovery'.[44]

Screening young athletes
A young life cut short is a devastating event for families, schools, sporting clubs and communities, and is associated with many lost productive years.[45]

Researchers at the Baker IDI Heart and Diabetes Institute in Melbourne consider SCA in the young to be a critical health issue and are endeavouring to learn more about its incidence and mechanism and the best strategies to prevent it. Sometimes there are symptoms like shortness of breath and fainting, or a person may have a family history of sudden cardiac death but many times, these deaths occur without warning. Although there is a lack of global consensus about the value of screening young athletes, Baker IDI aims to raise awareness of the issue and implement ongoing evidence-based research into the role of preventative cardiac screening.

Cardiologist and Director of Baker IDI Heart and Diabetes Institute Professor Garry Jennings says local health professionals and researchers are keen to understand whether screening of young athletes might prevent sudden deaths in the Australian setting.

Professor Jennings believes that cardiac screening of elite athletes would help researchers identify why there is increased danger and whether lives could be saved by more widespread screening.[46]

Italian authorities introduced screening for elite sportspeople when studies revealed that the SCA death rate among athletes with abnormal hearts rose from one in 100,000 for the general population to five in 100,000 for athletes who push their bodies to the limit. As part of periodic health evaluations (PHE), the European Society of Cardiology (ESC) and the International Olympic Committee also recommend pre-participation preventative screening to identify at-risk athletes.

Register for sudden cardiac death in young athletes

The rate of sudden cardiac deaths in young Australian athletes is not known and the Australasian College of Sports Physicians is one organisation that has advocated for an Australian registry to be established in order to determine the incidence and causes of these potentially preventable deaths.[47]

Training for families of young children

I have provided education and training on the use of an AED to the full range of age groups and demographics, young and old, male and female, including the parents and extended family of a five-month-old baby girl who could not go home from hospital until everyone caring for the child knew how to operate an AED. I have conducted training for the parents of a three-week-old baby boy who had survived a cardiac arrest at home and could not be discharged from hospital without a defibrillator. More recently, I have provided training for the parents and grandparents of a seven-week-old baby girl.

On separate occasions, I have also educated the parents, relatives, friends and childcare workers of a two-year-old boy, a three-year-old girl and a seven-year-old boy who must have an AED with them wherever they go. Two mothers of these children have the same genetic abnormality and are at risk of suffering sudden cardiac arrest themselves.

CASE STUDY: Kaydee Horne's family

What having an AED means to our family

The defibrillator for us is peace of mind, a way in which we can try and function as a 'normal' family. It is a resource that allows us to feel 'OK' leaving our daughter out of our care. People have a hard time comprehending what it is like to live with long QT syndrome, but the defibrillator and especially the training puts it into context. It makes us feel safe and it also makes our friends and family feel safe, as they will be forever worried and concerned regarding our condition.

To have AEDs available in the community would relieve a huge amount of anxiety, not only for me as a mother of a child with a cardiac issue, but also for myself, as I have the same cardiac condition. With so many people who are undiagnosed, I can also imagine the sense of relief for the community if they ever were confronted with someone in cardiac arrest. With the unpredictable nature of long QT syndrome, the defibrillator gives us hope that we might be OK and I would rest a little easier knowing that my daughter could have access to a defibrillator, wherever and whenever.

CASE STUDY: Jenny Whiteford's family

Education gave us peace of mind

Following our son's diagnosis of long QT syndrome (which he inherited from me), our anxiety was indescribable. We have had to live with the reality that our son could have a cardiac arrest at any time and, at this stage, he is too young to have a defibrillator implanted.

We recently purchased an AED and undertook a comprehensive training session with Anne Holland from Defib First, together with some family members and friends, in its use. Everyone who interacts regularly with our son is aware of his condition and what to do should he have an event, including how to use the AED. This minimises fear for us and them both in terms of looking after our son with confidence and potentially using an AED on anyone, anywhere, at any time.

The information, education and necessary skills we have all obtained are invaluable and have enabled us to push the diagnosis to the back of our minds, rather than it being in the forefront. Our son participates in the usual day-to-day activities of a toddler and is able to live his life to the fullest, radiating energy and personality. It is impossible to describe the immense relief and security we all now feel due to both having the unit on hand at all times and having absolute confidence in how to use it.

AEDs are becoming more prominent in society which is wonderful, but their presence is somewhat useless if members of the community don't have the knowledge and/or confidence to use them.

The purchase of our AED and the associated training session has resulted in numerous people gaining the important life skill of confidently using an AED. I am hopeful that many others will now do the same and have the potential to save a life.

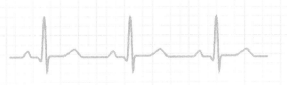

CHAPTER 8

THE CHAIN OF SURVIVAL

'Things do not happen, things are made to happen.'

JOHN FITZGERALD KENNEDY

The chain of survival refers to an internationally recognised series of actions designed to reduce the death rate associated with sudden cardiac arrest (SCA). It provides a critical timeline for rapid action before the arrival of paramedics or emergency medical services (EMS). If all of these steps are implemented quickly, the casualty has the greatest opportunity to recover and resume a normal life.

> Defibrillation is one crucial stage in a sequence of events that need to occur for the resuscitation of a victim of Sudden Cardiac Arrest (SCA). This sequence, or 'Chain of Survival', starts by summoning the emergency services as soon as possible. The second stage is providing basic cardiopulmonary resuscitation (chest compressions alternated with rescue breaths) to keep the victim alive until the third stage (defibrillation) can be performed.[48]
>
> *(Excerpt from Resuscitation Council (UK) and British Heart Foundation 2014 Guide to Automated External Defibrillators): Reproduced with the kind permission of the Resuscitation Council (UK)*

It is not well enough understood that recovering a victim at the scene of a cardiac arrest is just one of the critical elements in treating SCA. Obviously, though, if resuscitation is not successful at the scene, the rest of the links in the chain of survival become redundant. The victim's chance of long-term survival, and especially a return to normal life activity without any brain or cardiac deficits or complications, is directly proportional to the speed with which defibrillation occurs. The greater the delay in defibrillation, the less likely the victim will survive to be discharged from hospital even if they are successfully revived at the scene. It cannot be emphasised enough that *rapid defibrillation* is the key to survival – in the short and the long term.

For a successful resuscitation, the chain of survival requires the four 'Early'actions:

- Early access
- Early CPR
- Early defibrillation
- Early advanced cardiac life support

CASE STUDY: The chain of survival saves AFL doctor

A textbook example of the successful implementation of the chain of survival was the very public resuscitation of Dr Geoff Allen in July 2010. Geoff is one of the team doctors for the Geelong Cats Football Club in the Australian Football League (AFL). He was 48 years old when he suffered a cardiac arrest at AAMI Stadium in Adelaide on the field during the player warmup, prior to an AFL game (in front of the football crowd).

Medical and support staff swung into immediate action with early access, early CPR and early defibrillation within 90 seconds; Geoff was revived and waved to the crowd as he was carried from the ground and taken to the Queen Elizabeth Hospital in Adelaide.

Geoff had suffered a sudden cardiac arrest as the result of a heart attack and had there not been an AED applied so rapidly the outcome could have been much worse. During the fourth link in the chain of survival, advanced cardiac life support, a stent was inserted in a blocked artery in his heart within 20 minutes of his arrival at hospital.

Geoff has no cardiac impairment as a consequence of early implementation of the chain of survival and still runs, cycles and trains several times a week. He is also still a team doctor for the Geelong Cats.

Early access

The key to early access is witnessing the victim collapse or finding them without any delay, then phoning emergency medical services (EMS) immediately so that paramedics are dispatched and on their way, and managing bystanders and getting them to assist in the rescue. All of these actions enhance the likelihood of success.

Emergency calls can sometimes be inappropriately directed first to neighbours, relatives and local doctors. This causes delays and is associated with significantly poorer outcomes following out-of-hospital cardiac arrest (OHCA).[49]

The bystander's first phone call should always be to the EMS (in Australia, call Triple Zero (000)). Having EMS on the way immediately can have a significant impact on the effective and timely delivery of CPR and defibrillation and the arrival of medical help. Emergency operators will remain on the line to encourage and guide rescuers in CPR, which improves the victim's chance of survival from cardiac arrest.

When my husband, Paul, suffered a cardiac arrest, we did not find him early enough to be able to help him. He had a blockage in the same coronary artery (left anterior descending or LAD) which caused Dr Geoff Allen's cardiac arrest. Unfortunately for Paul, no-one witnessed his collapse. Without early access, it is virtually impossible to implement the remaining three actions in the chain of survival and achieve a successful outcome.

Early CPR

Cardio pulmonary resuscitation (CPR) is a critical step in the chain of survival and involves chest compressions and rescue breaths (*Cardio* = 'heart'; *pulmonary* = lungs). The most important component is effective chest compressions (PUSH HARD and PUSH FAST) with minimal interruptions.

CPR helps to sustain life by maintaining circulation of blood and oxygen to the vital organs: the brain and the heart. CPR is always performed because it buys time until an AED is applied or paramedics/emergency services arrive. It maintains an oxygen supply to the brain and keeps the heart muscle cells supplied with blood, preventing them from dying. Because it maintains perfusion (supply of blood and oxygen to the tissues), CPR also enhances the chance of survival once defibrillation is delivered. Perfusion increases the likelihood of the heart remaining in a 'shockable' rhythm rather than deteriorating to a 'non-shockable' rhythm (referred to in lay terms as a *flat-line*).

In Australia, the Victorian Ambulance Cardiac Arrest Registry (VACAR) data has shown that, in patients treated by emergency services, both survival at the scene of the arrest and survival to hospital discharge were significantly higher in patients who received bystander CPR compared with those patients who received no intervention from bystanders. Bystander CPR almost doubled in Victoria in the past decade, significantly increasing the likelihood of the victim still having an initial shockable rhythm when paramedics arrived. This is of critical importance because a victim of cardiac arrest is more likely to survive if their heart is in a rhythm that can be detected by the defibrillator as 'shockable' and which can then be reverted to a normal heartbeat by the shock from the defibrillator.

The presence of bystanders witnessing the arrest and/or providing CPR in public places has a significant impact on survival in these locations. A person who has a cardiac arrest in the workplace or a public place and receives bystander resuscitation is now three times more likely to survive long term than someone whose OHCA occurs in a private residence.[50]

Calling EMS immediately and delivering CPR promptly and effectively are crucial, especially for cardiac arrests that occur at home where defibrillators are not usually available. The priority in the early stages is to provide chest compressions, and if a rescuer is unable or unwilling to provide rescue breaths, then uninterrupted chest compressions should be given.

Early defibrillation

AEDs are automated, electronic defibrillating devices which are placed on the outside of the body (externally) and used to deliver a shock through the chest wall to reset the heart's electrical conduction system. However, too often an AED is not available or rescuers are too fearful to use it.

Defibrillation is the most vital and yet the most frequently missing link in the chain of survival. CPR buys time but on its own rarely saves a life.

Defibrillation is the only definitive and effective first aid treatment for SCA. A defibrillator delivers a lifesaving shock (electrical current) to the victim's heart, which restores life by stopping the abnormal chaotic electrical activity and allowing the heart to return to a normal rhythm or heartbeat. For every minute that passes without defibrillation, the likelihood of survival decreases by 9%–10%. The optimal time interval for defibrillation is within three to five minutes after a SCA and paramedics can rarely arrive that quickly.

In the 2014 *Guide to automated external defibrillators*, the Resuscitation Council (UK) and British Heart Foundation reinforced the importance of early defibrillation:

> The critical determinant of survival is the interval between collapse and the use of the AED to deliver a shock. The strategy, therefore, is to have an AED installed at a place where it might be needed so that it can be accessed quickly by someone nearby, taken to the person who has collapsed, and used before the arrival of professional help. This arrangement is known as Public Access Defibrillation (PAD).

> AEDs should be placed or stored where they are most likely to be needed; they must be accessible with the minimum of delay. All persons working at the site need to be aware of their purpose and location, and the steps to be taken should someone collapse.

> All that is required to use an AED is to recognise that someone who has collapsed may have SCA and to attach the two adhesive pads (electrodes) that are used to connect the AED to the patient's bare chest. Through these pads the AED can both monitor the heart's electrical rhythm and deliver a shock when it is needed. The AED provides audible instructions and most models also provide visual prompts on a screen.

> The AED will analyse the heart's electrical rhythm and if it detects a rhythm likely to respond to a shock, it will charge itself ready to deliver a shock. Some devices then deliver the shock automatically without needing any further action by the operator; others instruct the operator to press a button to deliver the shock (these are often referred to as 'semi-automatic' AEDs). After this the AED will tell the rescuer to give the victim CPR. After a fixed period (two minutes in current guidelines), the AED will tell the rescuers not to touch the victim while it checks the heart rhythm and a further shock is given (if it is needed). Using an AED in this way allows the provision of effective treatment

during the critical first few minutes after SCA, while the emergency services are on their way.[51]

(Excerpt from Resuscitation Council (UK) and British Heart Foundation 2014 Guide to Automated External Defibrillators): Reproduced with the kind permission of the Resuscitation Council (UK)

Early advanced cardiac life support

Anyone who has suffered a SCA, regardless of whether they have been revived by a defibrillator, must be transported to hospital for investigation, diagnosis and further treatment. On arrival at the scene, EMS or paramedics will take over treatment and management of the patient's condition and transfer them to specialised hospital care. Subsequent care includes intravenous access, administration of medications and other advanced cardiac life support (ACLS) techniques by emergency medical personnel, such as intubation (inserting a breathing tube into the airway) and oxygen administration. There is now significant evidence that hypothermia (lowering the patient's body temperature) enhances survival, with reduced risk of impaired heart and brain function. Cardiac arrest victims are routinely cooled in hospital now with the improved survival outcomes being due to low temperature slowing metabolic rate, the demand of the vital organs for oxygen and swelling of the brain.

It is vital for paramedics and hospital personnel to have a reliable history of the event. The AED stores critical data on heart rhythms, number and level of shocks delivered and time information which is useful later to medical staff for diagnosis and management of the underlying condition that caused the cardiac arrest. Survivors of SCA must have ongoing management by heart specialists (cardiologists and electrophysiologists) for follow-up care.

Part Three

THE IMPORTANCE OF DEFIBRILLATION

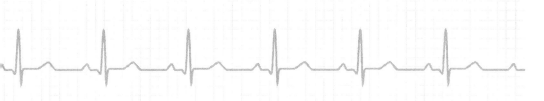

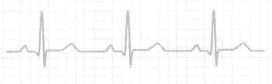

HISTORY OF DEFIBRILLATION TO PRESENT DAY TECHNOLOGY

'The things you do for yourself are gone when you are gone,
but the things you do for others remain as your legacy.'

KALU NDUKWE KALU

Defibrillation is based upon the understanding that contraction of the heart, and the resultant circulation of blood around the body, is under the control of an electrical conduction system specific to the heart. Electrical impulses generated by the sino-atrial node (SA node or pacemaker node) cause the chambers of the heart to contract regularly and rhythmically to pump blood into the circulation.[52]

The discovery that a misfiring heart could be restarted using an electrical charge is one of the great developments of modern medicine.

As early as Egyptian times

In an article for the University of Western Ontario Medical Journal, Stephen Chihrin described some fascinating facts about the early awareness of death caused by a trembling heart and later the effects of electricity on muscle cells. Chihrin wrote:

> The eminent danger posed by ventricular fibrillation was noted by the Egyptians as early as 3500 BC, when it was observed that 'When the heart trembles, has little power and sinks, the disease is advancing and death is near'.

The link between the heart trembling (fibrillation), having too little power (poor circulation), and death, was again described by physician Andreas Vesalius in the 1500s as 'worm-like' motions of the heart.[53]

18th Century discoveries

The discovery of electricity in the 1700s proved critical to research into heart function and defibrillation. The first reported case describing successful electrical shock resuscitation occurred in 1774, when a young female in England fell out a second-storey window and was believed to be dead. A doctor was eventually summoned and, after exhausting all conventional techniques, he attempted to apply electricity:

> *to various parts of the body in vain; but upon transmitting a few shocks through the thorax, he perceived a small pulsation (and) in a few minutes the child began to breathe with great difficulty, and after some time she vomited.*[54]

In 1775, Dr Peter Abildgaard published his observations on shock and counter-shock after he observed that electrical stimuli could, when applied anywhere across the body of a hen, and in particular the head, render his animal specimen lifeless, and that when electrical stimulation was applied again across the thorax, it could restart the heart:

> *With a shock to the head, the animal was rendered lifeless, and arose with a second shock to the chest; however, after the experiment was repeated rather often, the hen was completely stunned, walked with some difficulty, and did not eat for a day and night; then later it was very well and even laid an egg.*[55]

In 1791, Luigi Galvani made the classic observation that an electrical impulse could cause a frog's leg to twitch 'as though it were seized with tetanus at the very moment when the sparks were discharged'; however, it was mostly used to ensure that someone was really dead.[56]

19th Century theories

In 1850, Karl Ludwig applied current directly to a dog's heart and made it quiver.

In 1889, Scottish physician John MacWilliam published in the *British Medical Journal* his belief that ventricular fibrillation (VF) was the cause of sudden death in humans but he believed that it had not been identified in humankind because most cases of cardiac arrest occurred out of hospital, where the response time exceeded the duration of fibrillation. (This problem still exists today without public access defibrillators!)

In 1899, Federico Battelli and Jean Louis Prevost, two physiologists from the University of Geneva, Switzerland, found that weak electrical current could cause VF; however, a stronger current could stop VF in animals. (VF is the quivering of the main pumping chambers of the heart, which are called the ventricles.)

20th Century developments

1900–1950s

Early defibrillators
William Bennett Kouwenhoven's interest in the 1920's crossed between electrical engineering and medicine and his most enduring contributions to science came from his work in this area. His engineering focus was on high-tension wire transmission of electricity but he became interested in electricity's possible role in reviving animals. He knew that, when applied to the heart, an electric current could start it again.

During the 1920s and 1930s, research in this field was supported by the power companies because electric shock–induced VF killed many power utility line workers. In 1933, Donald Hooker, William Kouwenhoven, and Orthello Langworthy published the results of an experiment which demonstrated that an internally applied alternating current could be used to produce a countershock that reversed VF in dogs.

From 1928 through the mid-1950s, Kouwenhoven invented three different defibrillators: the open-chest defibrillator, the Hopkins AC defibrillator, and then the Mine Safety Portable. These were intended for use within two minutes of the start of VF and at least one required direct contact with the heart.

First successful human defibrillation

In 1947, Dr Claude Beck, Professor of Surgery at Western Reserve University, Cleveland, Ohio, reported the first successful human defibrillation. Beck's theory was that VF often occurred in hearts which were fundamentally healthy, in his terms 'hearts too good to die', and that there must be a way of saving them. Beck first used the technique successfully during surgery for a congenital chest defect on a 14-year-old boy who went into VF. The boy's chest was surgically opened and Beck applied a 60 Hz alternating current (AC) and was able to stabilise the heartbeat. The patient lived and the defibrillator was born.

As a result of studies done on accidental electrocution victims and funded by the Edison Power Company, Kouwenhoven and William Milnor demonstrated the first closed-chest defibrillation on a dog. Kouwenhoven and Drs James Jude and Guy Knickerbocker realised the weight of the defibrillator's paddles raised the animal's blood pressure. Based on this observation and with the addition of work done with rescue breathing by Dr Peter Safar, Kouwenhoven later developed cardiopulmonary resuscitation (CPR) techniques.[57] In 1957, Kouwenhoven and his team invented a non-invasive method of defibrillation which involved applying electrodes to the chest wall to deliver the necessary electric counter-shock.

In the mid 1950s, Paul Zoll used the ideas learned from Kouwenhoven and performed the first successful external defibrillation of a human using an AC defibrillator on a patient. The AC defibrillator was used successfully between 1956 and 1961.

1960s

AC to DC current

In 1960, Bernard Lown introduced the first direct current (DC) defibrillator after scientists discovered that DC defibrillators had fewer adverse side effects and were more effective than AC defibrillators

Portable DC defibrillators

In 1967, Drs Frank Pantridge (regarded as the father of emergency medicine) and John Geddes, from Royal Victoria Hospital, Belfast, launched the first mobile coronary care unit and demonstrated that a portable, battery-powered DC defibrillator could save lives. Their device, however, was cumbersome to operate and heavy to move. A lighter weight design needed to be developed.

The Belfast experience became an emergency care model for mobile coronary care units that was quickly adopted throughout the western world. The external device was subsequently manufactured and sold globally; however, the units could only be operated by trained personnel who were skilled in recognising lethal heart rhythms and manually applying the defibrillator paddles to deliver a shock. This was not of any benefit to the majority of cardiac arrests that occurred outside of a medical facility.[58]

1970s

Automated defibrillators for layperson use

There was a clear need to develop defibrillators that non-professional users with minimal training could operate to save lives. As improvements in electronics and computers became available these technologies were also applied to external defibrillators which were redesigned to automatically detect VF.

During the early 1970s, Dr Arch Diack and Dr W Stanley Welborn developed a portable unit called a cardiac automatic resuscitative device (CARD) that could diagnose a heart that was stopped or fibrillating and deliver an electrical shock capable of restarting it. The device, which later became known as Heart-Aid, was designed for temporary use by laypersons in emergency situations before professional care could be administered.

In 1978, the automated external defibrillator (AED) was introduced. This device was equipped with sensors that, when applied to the chest, could determine whether VF was actually occurring. If VF was detected, the device called out instructions to deliver an electrical shock. These automated devices greatly reduced the training required to use a defibrillator and have saved thousands of lives.

1980s

First AED
Professor John Anderson (1942–2012) who was head of bioengineering at the Royal Victoria Hospital, Belfast, (and later co-founder of HeartSine) collaborated with Dr Pantridge to develop the world's first truly portable defibrillator designed for use outside of the hospital. In 1980, Anderson filed one of the first patents for automatic recognition of VF. His algorithm, at the core of every AED in the industry today, provided the sensitivity and specificity necessary for the development of the first AEDs. In 1981, the first AED was developed in Northern Ireland and included a flat screen display, read out and recording facilities.[59]

Late 20th century into the 21st century

Adhesive gel pads
Two major changes occurred in recent decades. The first involved replacing the paddles which were manually held against the chest wall with adhesive gel defibrillation electrodes or pads that are placed directly on the patient's skin. These defibrillation pads are safer for rescuers, can be used by laypersons, and because they conform to the contours of the chest they are generally able to deliver the current more effectively to the victim.

Skin is a poor conductor of electricity and external defibrillators must be able to deliver sufficient electrical current to reach the heart through the mass of skin, hair and tissue. Therefore, an adhesive conductive gel must be used between the electrode and the patient. The gel forms a conductive bridge between the skin and the electrode, allowing better charge transfer. Without this conduction medium, the level of the current reaching the heart would be reduced and the skin may also be burned.

Monophasic to biphasic waveforms
The second major change in defibrillation has been the use of biphasic truncated (BTE) waveform. Until the late 20th century, the Lown monophasic waveform was the standard for defibrillation with most external defibrillation shocks delivered via paddles placed upon the patient's chest and the electrical waveform travelled in one direction

through the heart, giving a high-energy shock, up to 360–400 joules depending on the model.

Although successful defibrillation could be achieved, monophasic shocks could also cause increased cardiac muscle injury and in some cases resulted in second- and third-degree burns around the shock pad sites.

AEDs manufactured since 2003 use a BTE waveform to deliver two sequential lower-energy shocks of 120–200 joules by alternating the direction of the delivery of electrical current to the heart between the two electrodes (pads) placed on the skin. One shock cycle is completed in approximately 10 milliseconds. Because of the two-directional approach, the peak current required to convert the abnormal rhythm significantly decreases the energy level needed for successful defibrillation, and the efficacy of the shock is greatly enhanced.

It is generally accepted that the lower-energy waveform of biphasic defibrillation results in less myocardial (heart muscle) damage from the shock itself, less risk of burns, a reduced rate of complications and reduced recovery time. An additional advantage was a significant reduction in the weight of the machine.

The BTE waveform, combined with automatic measurement of trans-thoracic impedance (resistance to electrical current through the chest wall) is the basis for modern defibrillators. Approximately 40% of cardiac arrest patients who received a single shock from a monophasic defibrillator remained in VF. Most biphasic defibrillators, however, have a greater than 90% first-shock success rate, that is, normal heart rhythm is restored more effectively and efficiently.

In 1990, while playing polo at Warwick Farm, Sydney, wealthy businessman the late Kerry Packer suffered a cardiac arrest that left him clinically dead for at least six minutes. Luckily, an ambulance that happened to be carrying a defibrillator was in the area. Mr Packer was revived by paramedics using the defibrillator and he was then airlifted to St Vincent's Private Hospital, Sydney, where he underwent bypass surgery performed by the late Dr Victor Chang (an acclaimed pioneering cardiac surgeon who was tragically murdered in 1991).

At the time, it was uncommon for an ambulance to have a defibrillator on board – it was purely by chance that the ambulance that responded had one fitted.

After recovering, Mr Packer donated a large sum of money to the Ambulance Service of New South Wales to pay for equipping all NSW ambulances with a portable defibrillator (now colloquially known as 'Packer Whackers'). He challenged the then NSW Premier Nick Greiner: 'I'll go you 50:50', and the NSW state government paid the other half of the cost.

This was the beginning of the introduction of defibrillators into every ambulance in the country and many lives have been saved as a result.

Implantable defibrillation devices

A further development in defibrillation started in the late 1960s with the invention of the internal device, known as an implantable cardioverter-defibrillator (ICD), which was pioneered at Sinai Hospital in Baltimore in the United States of America by a team including Michel Mirowski, Stephen Heilman, Alois Langer, Morton Mower and Mir Imran, with the help of industrial collaborator, Intec Systems of Pittsburgh. Research commenced in 1969 but it was 11 years before the first patient was treated. Similar developmental work was carried out by John Schuder and colleagues at the University of Missouri.

The work was commenced against much scepticism even by leading experts in the field of arrhythmias and sudden death. There was doubt that the ideas would ever become clinical reality. In 1972 Bernard Lown, the inventor of the external defibrillator, even stated that he believed that patients repeatedly affected by VF were better off in a cardiac care ward being treated by drugs or surgery to correct blood flow in the heart than to receive an implanted defibrillator which was in his view 'an imperfect solution in search of a plausible and practical application'.

Despite the lack of financial backing and grants, the researchers persisted to overcome problems in the design of a unit which would enable detection of ventricular fibrillation (VF) or ventricular tachycardia (VT). The first ICD was implanted in February 1980 at Johns Hopkins Hospital by Dr Levi Watkins, Jr.

Initially ICDs were only implanted in those people who had already had a cardiac episode. The invention of implantable units has, however, been invaluable and lifesaving not just to regular sufferers of heart problems but also to those who have been diagnosed with a cardiac condition that pre-disposes them to a cardiac arrest, for example, genetic heart rhythm abnormalities. In particular, ICDs are likely to be implanted in younger people who survive a cardiac arrest and require their underlying condition to be monitored and treated by an internal device. ICDs are also often implanted in siblings/family members of people who have suffered a cardiac arrest, when they are found to have the same genetic condition. There are numerous case study references in this book to families who have required this preventative intervention.

An ICD can detect a life-threatening heart rhythm and defibrillate it before the victim collapses, loses consciousness and progresses to full cardiac arrest and death. This early defibrillation can not only save the victim from the medical emergency, trauma, complications and costs of a cardiac arrest, but also limits the potential damage caused to organs when tissues are deprived of oxygen during a full cardiac arrest.

When the electrical current is delivered to the heart via an ICD, far less energy is required as the shock is applied directly to the heart muscle and not through the skin, hair and outer tissue. So there is not as much resistance to the current and therefore greater likelihood of success and less risk of residual damage.

The future of AEDs

GPS-guided defibrillator drones

The most recent advancement in AED technology has been the development in The Netherlands of drones to rapidly and precisely deliver an AED to where it is needed.

An engineering graduate at Delft University of Technology, Alec Momont, has created a rapid-response drone to overcome the delay in arrival of an ambulance. For his master's degree project, Alec built a prototype of an ambulance drone containing a defibrillator, a camera, a microphone and speakers. The drone – an unmanned, autonomously navigating aeroplane – is able to fly at speeds of up to 100 km/h (60 mph), carrying a defibrillator to the emergency scene.

It is anticipated that the drones would be located at central dispatching points and controlled by a paramedic, via a livestream video and audio connection, in response to an emergency call. The drone finds the patient's location via the caller's mobile phone signal and, using GPS, the controller flies the drone to the scene then gives direct personalised instructions to people near the victim, using the drone's cameras and speakers. The defibrillator itself operates automatically once it is placed on the victim's chest. According to Momont, a network of AED drones could significantly improve the rate of cardiac arrest survival from 8% to 80%.

The drone can cut the average travel time from 10 minutes to one minute. It weighs 4 kg, can carry another 4 kg, and is equipped with features that could reduce the time for a cardiac arrest victim to receive lifesaving defibrillation. Momont explains:

> It is essential that the right medical care is provided within the first few minutes of a cardiac arrest. If we can get to an emergency scene faster, we can save many lives and facilitate the recovery of many patients. This especially applies to emergencies such as heart failure, drownings, traumas and respiratory problems, and it has become possible because life-saving technologies, such as a defibrillator, can now be designed small enough to be transported by a drone.[60]

> Some 800,000 people suffer a cardiac arrest in the EU every year and only 8% survive. The main reason for this is the relatively long response

time of the emergency services (approx. 10 minutes), while brain death and fatalities [start to] occur within 4 to 6 minutes. The ambulance drone can get a defibrillator to a patient inside a 12 square kilometre zone within one minute.[61]

The concept is exciting, however, the drone needs further technical development and legal issues need to be resolved. There are unsolved problems involving drones operating in urban environments out of sight of operators and requiring more than just GPS to navigate and detect obstacles, such as buildings and power lines, as well as landing a drone with spinning blades in the midst of panicking human rescuers.

Alec Momont envisions additional uses for his ambulance drones, including the delivery of oxygen masks to people caught in fires. There is also the potential use of drones carrying equipment over bodies of water to assist swimmers or boat users in difficulty. He hopes the device, which could cost less than US$20,000, might be available in five years and save hundreds of lives.[62]

Emergency AED towers

Emergency towers containing public access AEDs will soon be available in Australia and can be situated on street corners and in areas where high volumes of people meet and socialise.

The all-weather, fully monitored emergency towers and cabinets can build community awareness and confidence and will provide a *true public access AED* and emergency support system to anyone, anytime, everywhere.

The towers provide communication with local emergency services, enable rapid AED access and provide surety that the AEDs are appropriately maintained and ready for use.

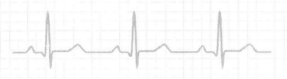

CHAPTER 10

HOW AEDS SAVE LIVES

'In the hands of those who get there first,
an AED provides the power to help save a life.'

CFA HEALTHWATCH AUSTRALIA

Sudden cardiac arrest (SCA) is the *one* cause of death which ordinary people can reverse before doctors or paramedics become involved. But unless bystanders step in and start the resuscitation, it's likely that the victim will die. If the victim does not survive at the scene of the cardiac arrest, the fourth link in the chain of survival, medical care in hospital, is no longer an option.

Automated external defibrillators (AEDs) provide essential, immediate and lifesaving treatment to someone suffering a SCA in the community. With increased public awareness and education and widespread availability of AEDs, the victim's chance of survival can be dramatically improved.

How awesome is that – to be an urban lifesaver and actually be responsible for reversing death and restoring a life!

The number of people who survive SCA is slowly increasing, thanks to bystander intervention with early cardiopulmonary resuscitation (CPR) and the early use of AEDs which are designed to be used by laypersons. The development of defibrillators that are easy to use has facilitated the growth of public access defibrillation (PAD), which experts agree has the potential to be the single greatest advance in the treatment of out-of-hospital cardiac arrest (OHCA) since the development of CPR.

CPR is critical during a cardiac arrest and must always be performed to give the victim the best chance of recovery because it buys time and maintains temporary perfusion (circulation of blood). But on its own, CPR is not enough. Defibrillation is the only effective first aid treatment to reverse cardiac arrest. The evidence is unequivocal that early defibrillation by first responders (members of the public) using an AED dramatically improves the casualty's chance of survival to over 80%. Without early defibrillation ideally within the first five minutes, usually less than 5% of people who have a SCA will survive in the long term.

Layperson or bystander rescuers can and do use AEDs in public areas until emergency medical assistance arrives. The AED gives an electric shock which stuns the heart, thereby stopping abnormal heart activity and allowing a normal heart rhythm to resume. If, however, bystanders do not act immediately or if there is a break in the chain of survival, it is unlikely that medical aid would make any difference.

Paramedics (traditional emergency responders) usually cannot arrive early enough to achieve effective and successful resuscitation resulting in the victim surviving in the long term. That means that some victims may be recovered at the scene and be transported to hospital but then do not survive to be discharged from hospital, due to complications related to delayed defibrillation.

Ambulance services in Australia are second to none and cardiac arrest will always be given immediate top priority. There are many variables, however, that can affect the ambulance response with arrival times for a Priority Code dispatch averaging around 10 minutes. Too often, paramedics arrive outside the optimal window of opportunity to revive the casualty. If bystanders act while the ambulance is on its way, the victim's chance of survival is dramatically increased.

Defibrillation explained

Contraction of the heart's chambers, and the resulting pumping or circulation of blood around the body, is under the automatic control of an electrical impulse which starts in the top of the heart at the sino-atrial node (SA node), known as the 'heart's natural pacemaker'. The electrical impulse moves down conduction pathways through the millions of cells of the heart muscle, causing it to contract or squeeze regularly, rhythmically and in a controlled sequence. The coordination of the pumping action is critical for the heart to function correctly.

Defibrillation is the definitive treatment for the life-threatening cardiac arrhythmias (disruptions to the electrical signals that control the contraction or pumping of the heart) which cause SCA.

The suffix 'de-' at the beginning of any word means 'to stop' or do the opposite or reverse. Hence de-fibrillation simply means reversing the lethal fibrillating rhythm by applying a therapeutic dose of electrical current or shock through the chest wall to the affected heart muscle cells. The shock momentarily stops the abnormal electrical activity, allowing the heart to re-establish an effective, regular and healthy normal rhythm. In simple terms, it is similar to turning off a light switch and turning it on again or using 'Ctrl-Alt-Del' to reboot a computer.

An AED is a portable electronic device that automatically detects and analyses heart rhythms and advises the delivery of a shock if the heart is in a shockable fatal rhythm or 'cardiac arrhythmia' (abnormal heartbeats) such as ventricular fibrillation (VF) and ventricular tachycardia (VT).

Circulation or perfusion of blood

As described in Chapter 6 'What is sudden cardiac arrest?', blood circulates or perfuses throughout the body of any living creature in a closed pumping or 'irrigation' system. The heart is the central pumping station which rhythmically contracts, pushing blood around the body under pressure. The pressure allows the blood to return to the heart to be recirculated, after it has been replenished with oxygen from the lungs. If the pressure drops, or stops all together (as occurs in a cardiac arrest) then blood circulation cannot be sustained.

Shockable heart rhythms

Normally, there is a brief time interval between one heartbeat and the next. During this interval (cardiac refill) the heart's chambers refill with blood ready for the next contraction. There are two types of 'shockable' cardiac arrhythmia: ventricular tachycardia (VT) and ventricular fibrillation (VF). In both VT and VF, the heart muscle is still electrically active but is in a dysfunctional state that does not allow the heart to contract and refill effectively in order to pump and circulate blood.

Ventricular fibrillation (VF)

VF is a lethal malfunction of the heart's electrical rhythm that occurs during a cardiac arrest. As previously explained, the term 'ventricular' refers to the lower chambers of the heart, the ventricles. 'Fibrillation' is chaotic electrical activity of the heart muscle cells which results in quivering rather than controlled and effective pumping. VF causes the heart muscle to lose its coordinated contraction, resulting in a dramatic drop in blood pressure so that the heart no longer pumps or circulates blood at all.

With the pumping activity of the ventricles no longer coordinated, the sudden loss of cardiac output and therefore blood pressure means there is no longer effective circulation of blood and oxygen. The vital organs, particularly the brain and the heart itself, are most susceptible to the loss of oxygenation, and without rescue intervention tissue death begins within minutes.

Anyone whose heart is in VF is clinically dead. Although VF is fatal, there is still electrical energy present. VF is an irregular fatal rhythm that can be reversed if an AED is applied quickly.

(Clarification: The term 'clinically dead' causes confusion. It does literally mean deceased; however, when used in the context of a sudden cardiac arrest, it refers to the victim being dead but there is the potential to be revived if resuscitation is commenced quickly. The victim will of course remain dead if there is no resuscitation.)

Ventricular tachycardia (VT)

VT is another abnormal cardiac rhythm that is shockable and can be reversed. VT can precede VF during a cardiac arrest. In VT, the ventricles of the heart contract or beat too fast to effectively refill the heart with blood between beats, so the heart cannot pump enough volume of blood out into the circulation. It is a little like an irrigation system – the pump is running but the water pressure is too low for adequate flow.

Ultimately, the heart muscle cannot keep up with such rapid contractions, weak blood pressure and low volumes of blood in circulation, all of which cause a drop in supply of oxygen to the heart muscle cells. VT is not sustainable over time. If it is not corrected, VT quickly progresses to VF which means the electrical activity of the heart 'virtually loses the plot' and becomes quivering and chaotic, preventing the ventricles (the heart's lower chambers) from effectively pumping blood.

Examples of VT & VF can be found in 'Chapter 6 – What is sudden cardiac arrest' (Figures 3 and 4).

How does an AED work?

When someone collapses from cardiac arrest, after rescuers call emergency services and start chest compressions, (after checking airway and breathing), it is vital that the heart is shocked back into rhythm with a defibrillator as soon as possible to increase the victim's chances of survival. Yet most people have never seen an AED and fewer still would know how to use one with confidence.

An automated external defibrillator is *external* because the rescuer applies the electrode pads to the outside of the victim's bare chest, as opposed to internal or implanted cardioverter defibrillators (ICDs). As described in Chapter 9 'History of defibrillation to present day technology', ICDs can be surgically implanted inside the body of a patient who is considered at risk of suffering a cardiac arrest. ICDs constantly monitor the patient's heart rhythm and activate automatically if the unit detects a life-threatening heart rhythm. ICDs usually defibrillate before the patient has progressed to a full cardiac arrest.

Automated refers to the AED's ability to autonomously (by itself) detect, analyse and diagnose the patient's heart rhythm and determine if a shock is needed.

Throughout a cardiac arrest, the SA ('pacemaker') node that stimulates the heartbeat continues to try to do its job and regain control of the heart rhythm but it can't break through the chaotic activity. If the heart can be shocked quickly with a defibrillator, within minutes of collapse and while there is still electrical stimuli (energy) present in the victim's heart, the abnormal energy ceases long enough for the SA node's signal to 'slip in', take over again and restore a normal heart rhythm.

In other words, defibrillation sends an electrical current through the heart muscle cells, which momentarily stops the abnormal electrical energy and reverses the lethal rhythm by allowing the SA node to resume normal activity. As mentioned earlier, this is similar to flicking a switch to reset the system.

Analyses the heart rhythm

All AEDs analyse the victim's heart rhythm and determine whether a shock is needed. AEDs can be either semi-automated or fully automated. A semi-automated AED uses voice prompts to advise that a shock is required and directs the rescuer to deliver the shock by pressing a flashing button. A fully automated AED delivers the shock after advising rescuers to stand clear and does not require the rescuer to take additional action (i.e. the rescuer does not need to push a button).

An AED cannot work unless it has detected a shockable, life-threatening cardiac rhythm. In other words, the AED controls if and when a shock is delivered and it will not operate indiscriminately. Both adhesive pads must first be applied to the patient's bare chest and then the AED must detect and analyse the victim's cardiac rhythm. It will only advise that a shock is required if it detects a shockable rhythm, that is, VT or VF. It will not deliver a shock if it detects a normal heart rhythm or a flat-line.

An AED cannot be used inappropriately nor will it inadvertently deliver a shock to the wrong person. Even if the button was pressed accidentally on a semi-automated AED, the device would not discharge any electrical energy if it was not necessary.

Gives automatic audio and visual commands

AEDs guide the rescuer with a very loud programmed electronic voice that prompts each step. Many AEDs also include visual display screens in case the rescuer has a hearing impairment or there is too much noise in the vicinity for the rescuer to accurately hear the instructions.

With automated audio and visual commands, AEDs are designed to be simple and easy for the layperson to use. Although AEDs are safe, in a perfect world laypeople should be trained and practised in operating them. Lack of prior training, however, should never prevent a rescuer from applying an AED.

What if 'no shock' is advised?

An AED will not tell the rescuer what kind of heart rhythm it has detected; it will only announce whether or not a shock is advised. If the AED advises 'no shock', it can never be assumed that a victim of cardiac arrest cannot be saved. Only someone who is qualified to make that decision, such as a paramedic or doctor, should do so.

If the victim is unconscious and not breathing, it is imperative to perform CPR until a defibrillator arrives and is applied to the victim and to continue CPR after each analysis by the AED until emergency medical services (EMS) take over care of the patient. It is, of course, acceptable to cease CPR if the victim starts to breathe normally, if there is imminent danger, or if the rescuer is exhausted and physically cannot continue and no-one else is able to take over.

How does a defibrillator reverse sudden cardiac arrest?

The AED's electrode pads are coated in a sticky, gel-like substance that provides a medium or pathway for conducting electricity from the AED into the victim's chest. The gel also adheres the pads to the skin for optimal delivery of the shock energy. The electrical current from a defibrillator is programmed to travel between the pads or electrodes through the victim's chest wall to concentrate the shock on the heart muscle.

Modern AEDs will discharge the electrical current in both directions (biphasic) between the two electrode pads on the chest, meaning that the current discharges from both pads and travels through the heart to the opposite pad. This is an improvement on past models because the biphasic waveform delivers less energy than was once required when the shock flowed only in one direction (monophasic). Using less energy means there is less risk of injury to the victim and less risk to others. Because the biphasic waveform flows in both directions, the electrode pads can be placed interchangeably on the chest; it doesn't matter which pad is placed on the upper right chest under the collar bone and which pad is placed on the lower left chest in line with the armpit – the shock will flow in both directions through the heart, regardless. With the pads being interchangeable, there is less hesitation and uncertainty when placing them on the chest, making the process simpler.

The pads are clearly marked with diagrams showing where to place them so it is highly unlikely that they will be applied incorrectly. However, even if the pads were placed on the opposite sides of the body, that is, on the *upper* left chest and *lower* right chest, the AED would still detect the victim's heart rhythm and would still deliver a shock if necessary. It is just not the ideal direction for the flow of the energy and the shock can be less effective.

After the rescuer applies the electrode pads to the casualty's bare chest, only then is the AED programmed to detect and analyse the electrical activity of the victim's heart. If the AED determines that the victim has a shockable, life-threatening heart rhythm, it will announce that a shock is advised and will warn bystanders to stand clear. The AED will then charge and deliver the shock through the electrode pads on the casualty's chest (a semi-automated AED will instruct the rescuer to press a button to deliver the shock).

A simple sporting analogy of how defibrillation works

The players in a team (*heart muscle cells*) erupt into a spontaneous melee causing disorganised, chaotic mayhem which stops the game (*normal heart rhythm*).

The team captain (*SA pacemaker node of heart*) tries to restore order and team cooperation but no one is paying attention.

The umpire (*defibrillator*) blows the whistle (*delivers a shock*) which stops everyone running amok and allows the team captain (*SA node*) to regain control of the players (*heart muscle cells*). The game (*normal heart rhythm*) can be re-established (*life restored*).

What if the AED detects a non-shockable rhythm?

A defibrillator cannot work unless it has detected an abnormal, shockable, life-threatening cardiac rhythm. If an AED was applied to someone and it detected a normal heart rhythm, the AED would not advise or deliver a shock.

Ventricular tachycardia (VT) and ventricular fibrillation (VF) are the most common, shockable rhythms during a cardiac arrest, but due to lack of blood pressure and insufficient circulation of blood to the vital cardiac tissues, if VT or VF is left untreated the electrical energy in the heart gets progressively weaker and fades out as the heart muscle cells die. If this happens, the victim's heart rhythm will quickly progress to *asystole* (pron. 'ay-sis-toe-lee'), popularly known as flat-line or cardiac standstill.

Once a heart that is in cardiac arrest reaches the point of flat-line, it is no longer possible for a defibrillator to administer a shock and restore a normal rhythm because there is no longer any electrical activity for the AED to detect and reverse. When flat-line occurs, the only chance of survival is a combination of CPR and cardiac stimulant drugs administered by paramedics in the hope of re-establishing a shockable rhythm.

If the AED is unable to detect a shockable heart rhythm or if it detects a normal heart rhythm, it will state 'no shock advised' and will not discharge any energy or shock. It is therefore not possible for an AED to shock someone who doesn't need to be shocked, or to inadvertently shock the wrong person, or to shock indiscriminately without warning (see Chapter 15 'Myth 3 – An AED can shock someone who doesn't need to be shocked').

Why is the time to first defibrillation so critical?

Without prompt intervention and resuscitation during a cardiac arrest, the abnormal rhythms (VT, VF and asystole) rapidly lead to irreversible heart and brain damage and death. The brain and tissue damage can begin to occur after approximately four to six minutes following the onset of cardiac arrest.

It is widely accepted that reducing delays before defibrillation begins leads to better outcomes for patients whose hearts are in shockable rhythms. The graph in figure 6 represents a cardiac arrest in which there is no intervention: no CPR and no defibrillation. For out-of-hospital cardiac arrest (OHCA) victims with a shockable rhythm, it is estimated that the likelihood of survival decreases by 9%–10% for each minute that defibrillation is delayed.

If there was no attempt at resuscitation, the heart muscle cells would begin to die and after 8–10 minutes of cardiac arrest, the electrical impulses would weaken and fade away, leaving no electrical activity at all. This is known as asystole (cardiac standstill or flat-line). The chances of recovering the victim at this point are extremely low.

Early defibrillation is critical to survival from sudden cardiac arrest for several reasons:

- When the event is out-of-hospital and witnessed, the most frequent initial rhythm is VF.
- The treatment for VF is defibrillation.
- The probability of successful defibrillation diminishes rapidly over time.
- Without defibrillation, VF deteriorates to asystole or flat-line.

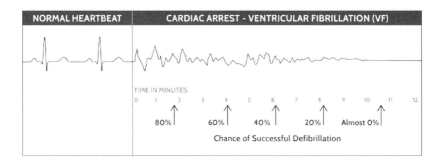

Figure 6. The chance of survival is greatest if an AED is applied
in the first five minutes.

When bystander CPR is provided, the survival rate decreases more gradually. On average, the survival rate with bystander CPR decreases by 3%–4% for every minute from collapse to defibrillation. If bystanders provide immediate CPR, many adults in VF can survive with intact neurological function, especially if defibrillation is performed within five to 10 minutes after onset of sudden cardiac arrest.

Basic CPR, alone, is unlikely to terminate VF and restore a perfusing heart rhythm, that is, a heart rhythm that delivers effective circulation; however, CPR does:

- prolong the electrical activity associated with VF and buy time
- delay the onset of asystole (flat-line)
- extend the window of time during which successful defibrillation can occur
- enhance the likelihood that defibrillation will be successful.

Even without access to a defibrillator, CPR must always be performed because it gives the casualty a chance at survival which is better than no chance. Sometimes there are good news stories despite a delay in defibrillation.

CASE STUDY: Sudden cardiac arrest survival at Montara Wines

In 2010, a 30-year-old member of our extended family, Michael Stapleton, was visiting his family's vineyard, Montara Wines in Victoria, for a meeting with their winemaker, Leigh Clarnette. During dinner, 53-year-old Leigh collapsed in cardiac arrest in front of his wife, Karen, and Michael, who had never had any first aid or CPR training; however, Karen had undertaken CPR training over many years in her role as a teacher and principal. Michael and Karen phoned Triple Zero (000) and were guided through CPR by the emergency operator.

The story had a very happy ending because paramedics were able to reach Leigh and defibrillate him, thanks to Michael and Karen's effective delivery of CPR, which maintained heart and brain perfusion of blood and oxygen until paramedics arrived. Despite requiring multiple defibrillation shocks in transport to hospital, Leigh survived and still works for Montara Wines as the winemaker.

Although this rescue finished with a successful recovery, it is not the norm because survival in these circumstances of delayed defibrillation is a most unusual albeit fortunate outcome. It is a lesson, however, that rescuers should always attempt and continue resuscitation until medical aid arrives because it can never be assumed that survival is beyond hope.

How do AEDs guide rescuers in providing CPR?

Apart from delivering a lifesaving shock, some AEDs also guide the rescuer in providing CPR. The Cardiac Science Powerheart G5 AED, for example, is programmed to assume that all rescuers do not know how to perform CPR. Therefore, after the AED has analysed the rhythm and, if needed, delivered a shock, it will automatically instruct the rescuer:

- Place heel of one hand on centre of chest between nipples.
- Place heel of other hand directly on top of first hand.

- Lean over patient with elbows straight.
- Press chest down rapidly one-third depth of chest then release.
- Start CPR.

The AED will set the rate and rhythm with a metronome beat (regular pinging sound) of 30 compressions followed by 2 rescue breaths. The metronome will ping to indicate each compression. After each cycle of 30 compressions, the AED will instruct:

- Stop compressions – give breath; give breath.
- Continue with 30 compressions.

It will repeat this cycle of 30 compressions and 2 breaths five times (or the equivalent of 2 minutes) before re-analysing the victim's heart rhythm.

It is critical for the victim's survival to avoid any unnecessary delays; therefore, if a rescuer *does* know how to apply an AED and perform CPR, the rescuer should bypass instructions from the AED and just get on with applying the pads and performing CPR if required. The AED will recognise which steps have been taken and will automatically progress to the next step.

Defibrillators used in hospitals and ambulances

Defibrillators carried on some ambulances and used in hospitals, and often seen on TV, are manual defibrillators. They are larger than AEDs, often have manual (handheld) paddles instead of adhesive pads, and are designed to be used by qualified medical personnel with specialised training who can recognise the heart rhythms and determine the electrical energy required for a shock, as well as when and how often to deliver it.

In contrast, AEDs are smaller, computerised and automated so that virtually any operator can use an AED by simply following the audio and visual prompts. The amount of energy and the decision to shock or not to shock is determined by the AED, not the operator.[63]

Quality control

Quality control of AED devices is stringent. Each company that manufactures medical devices, such as defibrillators, is required to register with the regulatory authority for the country in which they are being sold, for example, the Food and Drug Administration (FDA) in the United States and the Therapeutic Goods Administration (TGA) in Australia. Manufacturers must adhere to the quality standards known as 'good manufacturing practices' which require extensive record-keeping procedures. The manufacturer's facility can also be subjected to routine inspection of compliance to the standards. The majority of reported malfunctions are caused by failure to properly maintain defibrillators, rather than a manufacturing malfunction.

Maintenance

When I provide training sessions, one of the most common concerns about having an AED on site is 'what if the AED doesn't work when it is needed?' An AED is a machine, so there is always the unlikely possibility that an AED could be faulty. However, the risk of an AED malfunctioning is very low compared with the certainty that the victim will die if an AED is not available at all. These concerns should not prevent the acquisition of an AED.

Different AED models have different recommended maintenance schedules outlined in the user manuals. The manufacturer will specify how often the batteries and electrodes should be replaced. Good quality AEDs perform regular automated system checks and display rescue readiness or sound an alarm if there is any problem. It goes without saying that AEDs should always be maintained in a state of readiness. The most common reason why an AED malfunctions when it is needed in an emergency is not manufacturing errors but lack of maintenance checks and/or expired batteries and pads.

An AED that does not work properly when most needed will most likely be because the AED has been inadvertently overlooked and not monitored and serviced over the years.

CASE STUDY: When things go wrong ...

A non-working AED at a sports venue almost had tragic consequences.

In 2013 a family man in his forties was playing tennis at the Essendon Tennis Centre, Melbourne, when he suddenly collapsed on the court from a cardiac arrest. Luckily for him, an anaesthetist, Glen Burgin, and a fireman, Tony Devereux, also happened to be playing tennis and they immediately commenced CPR.

There was an AED on the premises of the tennis club but the battery was flat and it was inoperable. Someone with wisdom and foresight had installed the AED in good faith years earlier, but sporting clubs are volunteer organisations and members, volunteers and committees change over the years. Regulations do not exist yet to control the maintenance and safety tagging of AEDs as currently exist for fire extinguishers and electrical devices.

Fortunately, the adjacent Aberfeldie Sports Club had an AED and Tony De Fazio, who was also playing tennis that night, ran to the other pavilion, grabbed the AED off the wall and raced it back to the tennis club. The victim was revived with a shock from that device.

This rescue has special significance for my family. Our close and long-time friend Karen Rizzoli suffered a cardiac arrest in her sleep, six weeks before my husband Paul died in 2008. Following their deaths, Leigh Fotheringham, married to Megan, one of Karen's three daughters, installed an AED at Aberfeldie Sports Club.

It is a bittersweet irony that as a direct result of two tragic and unexpected deaths affecting our families and friends so close to one another, Leigh organised the purchase of an AED for his football club which then saved another person's life and enabled him to return to his family and resume a normal life. This is a wonderful gift and gives us much comfort.

The AED at the Aberfeldie Sports Club is registered and routinely monitored to ensure it is in working order with charged batteries and in-date pads. The tennis centre has since replaced their AED and I have provided their training. The AED is also regularly monitored on site and is registered with Ambulance Victoria's AED registry (www.registermyaed.com.au).

Monitoring

Although AEDs have audible alarms that sound when a malfunction occurs, they should still be monitored and checked at regular intervals to ensure that they are in rescue-ready mode at all times. Appropriate training and awareness including user checklists are critical for ongoing safe maintenance of AEDs. Monitoring and maintenance are discussed in greater detail in Chapter 11 'Public access defibrillation program'.

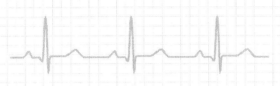

PUBLIC ACCESS DEFIBRILLATION PROGRAM

'The world hates change, yet it is the only thing that has brought progress.'

CHARLES KETTERING

Public access defibrillators (PADs) are also known as automated external defibrillators (AEDs). They are essential lifesaving equipment because they:

- provide the missing link in the chain of survival
- are automatic, safe to use and cannot be used inappropriately
- provide essential immediate and lifesaving treatment to a casualty suffering a cardiac arrest
- must first detect a *lethal* heart rhythm and *will not* deliver a shock indiscriminately
- *will not* shock someone with a *normal* heart rhythm
- are safe for anyone to apply during sudden cardiac arrest, regardless of prior training, and save a life by following the AED's voice prompts.

Technology has advanced to the degree that AEDs are safe for anyone to use regardless of whether they have had first aid training. If applied within the first few minutes after a cardiac arrest occurs, the shock from the defibrillator terminates the abnormal lethal heart rhythm and allows the heart's natural pacemaker to re-establish normal sinus rhythm (a normal heartbeat). This gives the victim a chance to live and to have the cause of their cardiac arrest diagnosed (and treated) in a hospital instead of at autopsy.

The Resuscitation Council (UK) and British Heart Foundation 2014 *Guide to automated external defibrillators* emphasises that AEDs are designed for and are safe for laypersons to use:

> AEDs are easy to use, compact, portable and very effective. Modern AEDs are very reliable and will not allow a shock to be given unless the heart's rhythm requires it. They are, therefore, extremely unlikely to do any harm to a person who has collapsed in suspected SCA. They are designed to be used by lay persons; the machines guide the operator through the process by verbal instructions and visual prompts. They are also safe and present minimal risk of a rescuer receiving a shock. They are designed to be stored for long periods without use and require very little routine maintenance or servicing; most perform daily self-checks and display/sound a warning if they need attention. Most AEDs currently offered for sale have a minimum life-expectancy of ten years. The batteries and pads have a long shelf-life, allowing the AED to be left unattended for long intervals.
>
> These features of AEDs make them suitable for use by members of the public with little or no training, and for use in PAD schemes. AEDs have been installed in many busy public places, workplaces, or other areas where the public have access. The intention is to use the machines to restart the heart as soon as possible. This strategy of placing AEDs in locations where they are used by lay persons near the arrest is known as Public Access Defibrillation (PAD). Training to use an AED is an extension of the first aid skills possessed by first aid personnel and appointed persons. AEDs have been used successfully by untrained persons, and lack of training should not be a deterrent to their use.[64]
>
> *(Excerpt from Resuscitation Council (UK) and British Heart Foundation 2014 Guide to Automated External Defibrillators): Reproduced with the kind permission of the Resuscitation Council (UK)*

Making AEDs accessible

As mentioned in Chapter 10 'How AEDs save lives', response times for most ambulances in Australia are sometimes greater than 10 minutes, which is outside the critical few minutes in which the casualty's life can usually be saved. It is possible for the victim to survive with only CPR and without early defibrillation, but the chances of survival are drastically reduced the longer that defibrillation is delayed.

The number of publicly accessible AEDs is steadily increasing but there are still insufficient units in the community and workplace to satisfy the three-minute accessibility threshold, that is, an AED needs to be situated no more than three minutes away to retrieve it because it takes another couple of minutes to get it back to the victim and apply the pads. Getting the AED takes precious time and most people are not aware of the importance of applying an AED within those first critical minutes. Until recent times, AEDs were generally either possessed only by trained personnel, who would attend incidents, or else they were public access units, which could be found in places where significant numbers of people gather, such as shopping centres, airports, casinos, hotels, and sports stadiums.

Nowadays, fire service vehicles and some police units carry an AED for officers to use as first responders before paramedics arrive. These AEDs have significantly improved survival rates for people who have had a SCA. Some areas even have dedicated community first responders who are volunteers tasked with keeping an AED and taking it to any victims in their area.

The location of a public access AED should take into account where groups of people gather, regardless of their age or the type of activity. Children and teenagers, as well as adults, may fall victim to sudden cardiac arrest.

Locating AEDs in the community

Suburban retail shopping strips provide favourable locations for AEDs. An AED can be positioned at one business, all other traders can be made aware of its location, and signs can be displayed on the shopfronts to let the public know where to find it. In a shopping area, one of the ideal locations for an AED is the local supermarket because it is usually open the longest hours and provides the greatest accessibility. This initiative has already been implemented in the United Kingdom, where the Asda retail chain has installed AEDs into every one of its stores, warehouses and offices. This approach is catching on in other parts of the world.

Multi-level and high-rise buildings are densely populated and problematic because they are more difficult for emergency medical services (EMS) to access quickly. In high-rise buildings housing hundreds (even thousands) of people, location of AEDs on designated floors or, even worse, just on the ground floor only creates confusion and major time delays caused by waiting for lifts, travelling to the AED location and then getting a lift back to the scene of the cardiac arrest. One solution would be to place AEDs in all elevators, which would facilitate faster access and save critical minutes for victims of cardiac arrest.

The number of devices in the community is growing as prices fall to affordable levels. One developing trend is the purchase of AEDs to be used in the home, particularly by those with known existing heart conditions.

To make them highly visible, public access AEDs are often brightly coloured and mounted in protective cases near the entrance of a building. When these protective cases are opened or the defibrillator is removed, some AEDs will sound an alarm to alert nearby staff. Some units have a back-to-base alert system when the AED is removed, however, opening the case and removing the AED does not necessarily summon EMS, so rescuers should never assume and should always phone EMS directly. In any situation when a rescuer sends for or uses an AED, the patient will be unconscious, which always requires an ambulance to attend and the call to EMS should never be delayed.

A recent Australian development could see AED emergency towers on street corners in the future, similar to schemes already in place overseas. These towers will provide ready access to an AED and have back-to-base monitored communication.

Improving survival rates of out-of-hospital cardiac arrest

Out-of-hospital cardiac arrest (OHCA) is the most significant cause of disability and death in Australia. Much of the burden of treatment associated with sudden cardiac death occurs before a patient even reaches the hospital. Bystander action in public places, including bystander CPR, is a key factor influencing overall rates of survival.

First aid training focuses on providing aid to the victim at the scene of injury or illness. Obviously recovering someone from cardiac arrest on the scene is the most important objective. But the majority of people do not realise that the earlier a victim is revived from a cardiac arrest, the less likely they will have complications or even die at a later time as a result of the collapse.

Recovering the casualty on the spot is the number one priority; however, we also want that person to survive to reach hospital, then to survive to be able to leave hospital and, just as importantly, to survive with a quality of life comparable to their lifestyle before cardiac arrest. Although survival rates for discharge from hospital are improving, the longer the delay in applying a defibrillator, the less likely that the victim's long-term outlook will be a good one.

It is widely accepted that reducing delays to defibrillation leads to better outcomes for victims in shockable rhythms. We know that the probability of survival from OHCA is estimated to decrease by 9%–10% for each minute that first defibrillation is delayed. The most important and effective strategy for decreasing time to defibrillation is for bystanders to perform defibrillation using an AED.

Increase in bystander use of AEDs

Improvements in survival outcomes are supported by over a decade of growth in community-initiated CPR. The likelihood of survival is strongly associated with the presence of bystander CPR.

In February 2014, a media release from the Victorian Minister for Health and Ageing, David Davis MLR, based on statistical evidence provided by Ambulance Victoria, revealed that more bystanders than ever were recognising cardiac arrests and providing lifesaving resuscitation before paramedics arrived, greatly improving the victims' chances of survival. Use of AEDs by members of the public on cardiac arrest patients had increased from 1% in 2003–04 to 10% in 2012–13.[65] As a result, the proportion of patients surviving cardiac arrest and being discharged from hospital rose by 12% during that time. There are many Victorians alive today who owe their lives to bystander volunteers as well as paramedics.

The minister encouraged as many people as possible to receive basic training in CPR and in the use of defibrillators, which are real lifesavers when a cardiac arrest occurs.

Victorian Ambulance Cardiac Arrest Registry

In December 2014, Ambulance Victoria released the Victorian Ambulance Cardiac Arrest Registry (VACAR) report, which was even more encouraging of PAD programs. The VACAR was established in 1999, and represents an internationally recognised standard of OHCA monitoring and reporting. Data for all cardiac arrest patients attended by Ambulance Victoria since October 1999 (over 75,000 patients) has been successfully recorded. This program has resulted in the capture of data for almost 99% of all victims of OHCA transported to an emergency department in Victoria.

The VACAR report supported the American Heart Association view that monitoring and recording emergency medical services management and treatment of OHCA victims could provide the most valuable database of information which would lead to improved outcomes.

Survival rates with early defibrillation

The findings of the VACAR report are that cardiac arrest patients who receive early defibrillation by community members are approximately three times more likely to survive than those who have to wait for paramedics to arrive with a defibrillator.

A timely response by first responder teams and early intervention by bystanders remain key factors driving favourable outcomes for patients with shockable rhythms in Victoria. In fact, the proportion of cases where Ambulance Victoria performs the first defibrillation has reduced by 10% in recent years, from 91% in 2004–05 to 82% in 2013–14. There is a direct relationship between this reduction and a 10-fold increase in the use of public AEDs by bystanders over the same period.[66]

In 2013–14 the outcomes for patients receiving first defibrillation by bystanders were particularly rewarding. First defibrillation occurred sooner in cases where bystanders applied an AED (5.2 minutes) compared with waiting for paramedics (10.0 minutes). The proportion of patients who survived cardiac arrest when first defibrillated by a public AED was 64% compared with 53% who were shocked by paramedics and 57% who were shocked by first responders (such as police or fire brigade).

The likelihood that a victim would survive to hospital discharge also differed significantly depending on who provided the first defibrillation. Victims who were defibrillated by a bystander using an AED were 62% more likely to survive to hospital discharge compared with victims whose first defibrillation was provided by EMS.

Survival rates with early effective CPR

Previous research by VACAR had shown that early effective bystander CPR increased the likelihood that the victim will have an initial shockable rhythm, and greatly improved the victim's chance of survival following OHCA.[67] Over the past decade in Victoria, there have been significant increases in rates of bystander CPR. In cases where bystanders witnessed a person collapse in sudden cardiac arrest, the chance of the victim receiving CPR from bystanders was 61% in 2013–14, compared with 35% in 2004–05.

In the cardiac arrest population who were still in a condition that was treatable when paramedics arrived, both survival of the event and survival to hospital discharge were significantly higher in those patients who received bystander CPR compared with those who received no intervention from bystanders.

Further outcomes

Other outcomes from the VACAR report are:

- Less than 10% of bystander calls for help following OHCA are inappropriately directed to a relative, friend or neighbour rather than directly calling for an ambulance.
- In 2013–14, EMS were able to continue resuscitation in 75% of OHCA cases where bystanders had started CPR prior to EMS arrival compared with only 43% of bystander-initiated CPR in 2004–05.

- In 2010, VACAR became one of few registries around the world that routinely captures the quality of life of adult survivors of OHCA at 12 months after the event. 84% of OHCA survivors (2013–14) with known survival to be discharged from hospital maintained their independence and had a good quality of life 12 months after their cardiac arrest.

Associate Professor Karen Smith, VACAR principal investigator and chair, stated that:

> Our research agenda focuses on every aspect of the Chain of Survival, from the early actions of bystanders and EMS following patient collapse to outcome at hospital discharge. We continue to strive towards addressing the important and unanswered questions relating to cardiac arrest. More widespread availability of AEDs in public places may further improve OHCA survival.[68]

As the evidence gathers, it is becoming clear that AEDs are making a significant difference – increased awareness has resulted in rescuers looking for an AED and using it before paramedics arrive. More widespread availability of AEDs in public places is leading to improved OHCA survival.

CASE STUDY: Jenny Gifford's rare survival

Jenny Gifford's story of survival helps to illustrate the success of public access defibrillation but also highlights the potential for medical complications when defibrillation is delayed.

On 14 October 2013, Jenny Gifford, a 51-year-old mother, was playing basketball at St Arnaud in Victoria when her heart suddenly stopped and she crashed to the court. Bystanders immediately commenced CPR but the St Arnaud ambulance was attending another call and the next closest ambulance was 30 minutes away. There was, however, a public access defibrillator 2 km away at the local netball club. CPR was continued and kept her well perfused, but due to the distance travelled to retrieve the AED there was a considerable delay to first defibrillation. The AED was retrieved and bystander rescuers used it to defibrillate Jenny approximately 15 minutes after she collapsed.

Despite the rural location, emergency medical services swung into action with seamless precision. After she was defibrillated at the scene by bystanders, followed by arrival of paramedics, the air ambulance helicopter airlifted Jenny to the Alfred Hospital in Melbourne where she was maintained in a medically induced coma for 11 days. Jenny had multiple cardiac arrests; however, her good news story is a very fortunate one because although her remarkable recovery was not without medical complication (in that she needed to be kept in a coma for so long and she arrested more than once), she has survived to resume her normal life without any neurological deficit. She now has an implanted defibrillator and the cause of her cardiac arrest is unknown. It was not a heart attack as most would assume.

More often than not, with such a long delay to defibrillation, the survival outcome is not so positive. Associate Professor Tony Walker, Ambulance Victoria's general manager of regional services at that time, said Mrs Gifford's survival was a perfect example of citizens doing a great job in early CPR and defibrillation to support paramedics' work in regional areas:

> Ambulance services in the country actually start with the community and with the proliferation of automatic defibrillators and people with CPR training, communities can play an important role in caring for each other until the ambulance arrives.

Author's note: Jenny survived because community members took ownership of saving her life and despite the delay in getting an AED, they did not give up. It should also always be remembered that property is replaceable. If access to an AED is ever obstructed, damage to physical barriers can always be repaired later and should not prevent action necessary to save a life that is not replaceable.

Overseas experience

Europe

Studies in Europe support the VACAR findings. In recent years, wider use of AEDs to treat OHCA was advocated in The Netherlands after a seven-year study of OHCA. The findings concluded that between 2006 and 2012 there was a significant increase in rates of survival with good neurologic outcome (brain function) after OHCA in patients with a shockable rhythm.[69]

Survival increased at each stage of the resuscitation process, but the strongest improvement was noticed in the prehospital (at the scene) phase. Rates of AED use almost tripled during the study period, which meant the time from emergency call to defibrillator connection was decreased. Increased use of AEDs is associated with increased survival in patients who were defibrillated by an AED. Ongoing efforts to improve resuscitation outcomes were recommended with strong emphasis on introducing or extending public access and first responder AED programs.[70]

PRNewswire reported in February 2015 on an analysis and forecast of revenue estimated for the European automated external defibrillators (AED) market which is estimated to grow to about US$134.2 million by 2019, at a compound annual growth rate of 10.9% from 2014 to 2019. The major drivers behind the growth and distribution of AEDs in Europe are the increasing rate of cardiovascular diseases, government regulations regarding PAD and advances in technology.

Italy and France passed legislation in 2001 and 2007 respectively, authorising the use of AED by a layperson. As a result of these laws and nationwide defibrillation programs undertaken by various local and national governments, a large number of AEDs have been installed at public places such as shopping centres, airports, offices, government buildings, schools, health and sports clubs, transportation centres, day care centres and casinos. Thus, the increasing installation of public access AEDs boosts the growth of this market.[71]

United States of America
An editorial published in the American Heart Association journal *Circulation* on 18 November 2014 acknowledged the significant improvement in survival from cardiac arrest over the recent decades if there is immediate recognition and treatment with prompt implementation of the chain of survival. Early notification to EMS to get help on the way, bystanders starting CPR and applying an AED before EMS arrive and access to specialised medical care are the key predictors of a successful recovery.

In an article written in OH&S Online, 1 February 2015, Jim Madaffer (co-founder of San Diego Project Heartbeat) asked the question, 'Why don't we see more AEDs?' He wrote that:

> Having an Automated External Defibrillator (AED) nearby when SCA strikes increases the survival rate by nearly 70 percent …

> While fire extinguishers are required everywhere, most paramedics and firefighters will tell you they've used an AED far more often than a fire extinguisher.

> Despite slow deployment, these lifesaving devices are gaining more steam and seeing more support across the country. Some state and city governments now require the placement of AEDs, while others have passed laws protecting AED owners and enablers. Travelers see them in airports and more frequently in government buildings and businesses. The tide is turning to the point that not having an AED could result in potential liability.[72]

What if the AED is not working?

By far the most important maintenance task associated with AEDs is monitoring the 'rescue-ready' status over time. There are no regulatory requirements in Australia for monitoring, testing and tagging of AEDs, which are useless if the battery charge has expired and/or the electrode pads have dried out. Unsuccessful rescues have occurred with victims of cardiac arrest because the AED that was on site had not been routinely monitored or serviced and it was inoperable when it was needed most.

The story of an inoperable AED at a sporting club (Chapter 10 'How AEDs save lives') is a cautionary tale about the essential need to maintain AEDs in working order. If a working AED had not been available in that situation, the outcome could have been tragic.

Planned maintenance

It is imperative that AEDs are maintained in ready mode. Different AED models have different recommended maintenance schedules outlined in the user manual. The manufacturer will specify how often the batteries should be replaced. Many currently available defibrillators have regularly scheduled automated self-tests and display their operational status.

Monitoring logs and user checklists should be used to reduce the chance of equipment malfunction and operator errors.

Every checklist should include:

- a monthly check that the battery power indicator is green, designating adequate charge
- expiry dates of electrodes
- condition and cleanliness of the unit
- provision of adequate supplies such as personal protective equipment (PPE) – gloves, mask, scissors, disposable razor, paper towel
- replacement of consumables where indicated.

The electrode pads are single-use only so must be discarded and replaced after use. It is important to make sure that the pads stored with the AED are in date. If the conductive gel on the pads has dried out, the pads cannot be used. All manufacturers mark their electrode pads with an expiry date, and it is important to ensure that they are always in date. On some models the date is visible through a window, while for other models the case must be opened to check the expiry date.

Regulatory requirements

Depending on the size of the building, all public and workplaces must have fire protection equipment, which is at the very least, fire extinguishers. The 2012 Australian Standard AS1851–2012 – *Routine service of fire protection systems and equipment* mandates six-monthly inspection and tagging of fire extinguishers and other fire protection systems and equipment to ensure they meet the requirements of the relevant design, installation and commissioning standards and are likely to continue to do so until the next scheduled inspection. Despite regulations that require electrical equipment and fire extinguishers to be periodically tested and tagged, at the time of publication, there are no such regulatory requirements for monitoring the working order of AEDs, which are more likely to be used than fire extinguishers.[73]

Locating the nearest public access defibrillator

In Victoria, emergency services Triple Zero (000) operators have access to a centralised voluntary registry, Register My AED, where the location of AEDs in the community can be listed (see www.registermyaed.com. au). If a sudden cardiac arrest occurs at the address of a registered AED, an emergency operator can direct the caller to the location of the AED. This type of registry needs to be expanded to an integrated national and international service because currently there are multiple services which result in an incomplete and fragmented database. Privacy laws also prevent all AED locations from being shared.

Mobile phone apps

Mobile phone apps such as PulsePoint and GoodSam enable community first responders to register their availability to respond to a cardiac arrest in their vicinity. Volunteers are notified by SMS when an emergency occurs and if they are able to respond, the app notifies them of the location of the casualty and the nearest AED. In Japan, a free GPS-based app called Heart Rescue has been trialled to alert people who are trained in CPR that there is a cardiac arrest nearby. Widespread awareness of and participation in these services is not yet achieved which, therefore, limits their usefulness.

Training enhances the success rate of PAD programs

The availability and accessibility of public access defibrillators are fundamental components of successful rescue for cardiac arrest victims. One of the most common inhibitors that prevents members of the public from applying an AED is fear due to lack of understanding. Chapter 12 'Why are education and training so important?' will focus on education and regular refresher training for staff and members of the public, which can significantly improve survival outcomes.

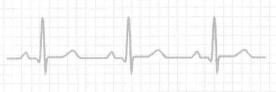

WHY ARE EDUCATION AND TRAINING SO IMPORTANT?

'Knowing is not enough; we must apply.
Willing is not enough; we must do.'

JOHANN WOLFGANG VON GOETHE

Organisations that provide training in CPR and defibrillation play an important role in busting the myths associated with AEDs and in giving laypersons the confidence to use an AED in an emergency. The perceived risk of doing 'more harm' and the fear of litigation are both common misconceptions among the general public and the private sector. Unfortunately these misconceptions are significant barriers to the use and uptake of AEDs, both in Australia and overseas. While it is important to understand that none of these myths are valid, the reality is that a trained person is more likely to have the speed and confidence to use an AED decisively, when an emergency situation demands it.

Education is the key to empowering ordinary people to become urban lifesavers. As people become more familiar with AEDs, and as there is more awareness within the community that it is safe (for both the victim and the layperson rescuer) to use an AED, bystanders will have the confidence to act as first responders. Early CPR and defibrillation give the best chance of survival and bystanders are best placed to provide that chance. Urban lifesavers know what to do and can act quickly to ultimately reduce the time to defibrillation. I repeat once again, sudden cardiac arrest (SCA) is the *one* cause of death that a bystander can reverse, if they act without delay.

Support from heart health organisations

According to Ambulance Victoria data, approximately 6,000 sudden cardiac arrests occur in Victoria each year. In a 2014 media release, Heart Foundation Victoria CEO Diana Heggie commented that defibrillators are an important part of the response to cardiac arrest and that community education is needed so Victorians have the confidence to use defibrillators. Ms Heggie said:

> It is a medical emergency that requires an immediate life-saving response ... Whilst evidence shows that lives can be saved when defibrillators are available in public places, members of the public must have the knowledge and confidence to use a defibrillator. Community education should also highlight the importance of calling 000 for an ambulance straight away. The sooner ambulance paramedics arrive on the scene the greater the chance of survival.[74]

The Resuscitation Council (UK) and British Heart Foundation 2014 Guide to Automated External Defibrillators reinforces this view:

> It is vital that as many people as possible learn basic skills in cardiopulmonary resuscitation. This entails recognising that someone may have suffered SCA, calling the emergency services and then performing chest compressions and rescue breaths. This basic first aid will maintain an oxygen supply to the brain and other organs and make it more likely that the heart can be re-started by defibrillation. The priority in the early stages is to provide chest compressions, and if a rescuer is unable or unwilling to provide rescue breaths uninterrupted chest compressions should be given.

> *Reproduced with kind permission of the Resuscitation Council (UK)*

The Australian 2012 *Joint statement on early access to defibrillation* called on the Australian, state and territory governments to support early access to defibrillation by building community confidence in the use of AEDs through the implementation of community awareness campaigns that highlight both the misconceptions and benefits of prompt AED use. (Appendix A.)

When someone collapses from cardiac arrest, the victim's chance of survival depends on how quickly their heart is shocked back into a normal rhythm with an AED. Yet most people have never seen an AED, other than on television, and fewer still would know how to use one with confidence and without fear. Breaking down the barrier of fear is difficult and depends upon correct information and education.

Movies, TV and myths about AEDs

The closest most people have come to seeing a defibrillator in action is watching their favourite medical drama. How many times do we see, in movies or on TV, the patient sitting up in a hospital bed, connected to a monitor with a beeping heartbeat spiking across the screen. Suddenly, the patient grasps their chest, passes out and goes into flat-line or cardiac standstill (the medical term is *asystole*). A doctor (wearing the stereotypical white coat) rushes in, grabs the defibrillator paddles, shouts 'clear' and zaps the patient's chest through the fabric of the gown. After a dramatic pause, the patient miraculously regains consciousness, sits up and orders dinner or prepares for discharge!

The Hollywood imagery bears no resemblance to reality but does give birth to mythology because it creates the impression that a cardiac arrest is a heart attack and has symptoms (myth), that someone can be defibrillated through clothing (myth), that the patient can be revived with a defibrillator when their heart has gone into flat-line (myth) and that only medically trained personnel can operate defibrillators (myth). As a result, layperson bystanders often believe that there is nothing they can do and that they must wait for more qualified responders to arrive.

The necessity for training and retraining

There is a frighteningly common presumption in the general population that having done a first aid course at some stage in the past qualifies one as first aid trained for evermore! Most people do not understand that their cognitive skills and thought processes can be significantly impaired when they are confronted with a medical emergency because the consequent adrenaline rush can create fear, confusion and anxiety in the bystander rather than decisive and beneficial action. It is only when training is regularly repeated and reinforced that the brain is able to recognise, focus and respond quickly and logically to an emergency. Critically valuable time can be lost if a rescuer becomes agitated or flustered, is unable to think clearly and cannot remember skills learned long ago.

All emergency services responders such as paramedics, firefighters, police officers, State Emergency Service personnel and medical and nursing personnel do their initial professional training and then continually update and refresh their skills. They practise, train and retrain because familiarity, reinforcement, repetition and rehearsal are best practice and the only way to remember what to do without delay in an emergency. Healthcare professionals must submit and keep records of annual continuing professional development and show evidence to maintain their registration and accreditation.

Even if AEDs are made more accessible and an increasing number are available, there is no guarantee that they will be used effectively. Time is of the essence in cardiac arrest and there is a risk that untrained rescuers will lack the confidence to use an AED when necessary. Those who do use it may hesitate or act slowly, which wastes valuable time and can cost lives. The more people who have the knowledge and the confidence to use an AED, the greater is the likelihood that resuscitation will be successful.

The Japanese Government made 350,000 AEDs available around the country in the last decade but although they are a common sight, they are rarely used due to lack of training. School children are now being taught how and why to use them.

The International Liaison Committee on Resuscitation (ILCOR) – Consensus on Science and Treatment Recommendations issued the following advice in 2010:

1. An AED can be used safely and effectively without previous training. Therefore, the use of an AED should not be restricted to trained rescuers. However, training should be encouraged to help improve the time to shock delivery and correct pad placement.

2. Short video/computer self-instruction courses, with minimal or no instructor coaching, combined with hands-on practice can be considered as an effective alternative to instructor-led BLS and AED

courses. Such courses should, however, be validated to ensure that they achieve equivalent outcomes to instructor led courses.[75]

Reproduced with kind permission of the Resuscitation Council (UK)

Australian, state and territory governments are urged to take a leadership role in raising awareness within the community on the importance, benefits and misconceptions of AED use and to legislate to bring the laws in line with current training regulations which were revised in 2013.

Legal protection for rescuers

Although training in the use of an AED is highly recommended for familiarity and confidence, an AED will deliver a shock *only* if it is deemed necessary (when it detects a shockable rhythm), so it is easy and recommended for laypersons, with or without prior training, to operate an AED in the event of a cardiac arrest.

Jurisdictions within Australia and many other countries have 'Good Samaritan' legislation in place which protects lay rescuers from the risk of litigation when they act in good faith in an emergency. Australian Good Samaritan legislation is listed in Appendix C.

Someone providing first aid should give emergency care that is:

- within the best interest of the victim
- prudent and reasonable in the circumstances
- provided in 'good faith', without recklessness and with reasonable care and skill
- in accordance with first aid principles and the level of skills and knowledge acquired during any previous first aid training
- unlikely to make the victim's condition worse, or complicate the illness or injury.

In a situation involving cardiac arrest, it is simply not possible to make the victim's condition worse because they are dead and without CPR and defibrillation they will remain dead. Furthermore, there have been no cases within Australia where a person or business has been sued for using an AED in a medical emergency situation.

Creating confidence to use public access AEDs

Public access AEDs are electronically programmed to automatically detect heart rhythm once the pads have been applied to the chest. The AED will deliver instructions and respond to rescuer hesitation by repeating instructions if necessary. Some models start issuing instructions as soon as the lid is opened and others have an on/off button. With all models, the decision to deliver a shock to someone is effectively taken out of the rescuer's control – if the AED does not detect a rhythm that will respond to a shock (a shockable rhythm), then it simply won't deliver a shock. All the rescuer needs to do is follow the instructions, apply the adhesive electrode pads, and either push a button when prompted or allow the device to automatically deliver a shock.

Addressing myths and fears

AEDs are simple and easy to use and are programmed with clear voice instructions for the rescuer to follow. The user cannot override an AED and deliver a shock manually. But having AEDs available for laypersons to use is only helpful if people are confident to use them without the inhibitions created by myths and fears.

In my experience as a trainer and presenter, rescuers who are fearful are unlikely to 'have a go' regardless of how easy the unit is to apply! So, it is critical to properly educate and instil confidence in the general public (non-traditional responders)[76] to use AEDs and provide resuscitation. However, skills degrade rapidly without repetition and rehearsal.

Maintaining knowledge and skills

There is no point having an AED if not enough people know what to do with it, so regular ongoing updates and refresher training are just as important as the initial training. The evidence supports that low-dose, high-frequency refresher training doubles the learner's capacity to retain what they have learned. The services provided by Defib First of one-hour information presentations deliver sufficient knowledge to instil confidence and are ideal for meeting the low-dose, high-frequency training criteria.

Being prepared

Time and time again, I attend venues and organisations to deliver an information and demonstration presentation on how and why to use an AED, only to find that the staff or members have not even opened the delivery box because they don't know what to do with it or are too fearful to touch the AED in case they do something wrong or injure themselves or someone else. On one occasion, the AED had been on display in its wall bracket and fully accessible for a couple of months without the battery in it. Had there been a cardiac arrest incident, the AED would have been useless.

The frontline motto of the Australian Resuscitation Council is: *Any attempt at resuscitation is better than no attempt.* The truth is, it is not possible to harm someone who is in cardiac arrest because they are dead and AEDs cannot be used inappropriately; they are safe, reliable and effective. AEDs *work*!

AED information training sessions by Defib First

The one-hour information presentation provided by Defib First focuses not only on how the AED operates, but just as importantly, explains what a cardiac arrest is, what type of heart rhythm an AED is looking for, what sort of rhythms it can shock and why it is so vital to provide that shock quickly.

At the beginning of my Defib First information session, I often suggest the scenario of standing at the baggage collection carousel of an airport (where AEDs can be found on the nearby walls). I ask the attendees: if they witnessed the person beside them at the carousel collapse and stop breathing, would they have the confidence to grab the AED off the wall and apply it to the casualty's bare chest?

The attendees are requested to mark their responses as follows:

Prior to today's presentation, would you feel confident to apply an AED to a casualty?

a) Yes, without hesitation
b) Yes but only if a more qualified person instructed me

c) Don't know
d) No

The presentation is delivered in an easy-to-understand format. Although some of the information is technical, it is understandable and it is not necessary nor is it expected for those in attendance to remember all the detail. The goals of the presentation are to give enough explanation so the attendees understand what cardiac arrest is and how to recognise it, and to give them the confidence to apply an AED. The presentations empower laypeople to become urban lifesavers and potentially save a life. At the same time, they are reassured that they can do no harm, nor can they be held liable.

Medically trained persons sometimes hold an arrogant belief that the 'average Joe' layperson cannot possibly understand medical terminology and physiology. My experience from presenting these information sessions to the lay population couldn't be further from that viewpoint.

At the conclusion of the presentation, I usually revisit the scenario of the airport baggage carousel and ask the question again: Would you grab the AED off the wall and use it? The responses from the 'before' and 'after' questions are always very different and gratifying and are indicative of the importance of this type of education.

Prior to the presentation, 90%–95% of respondents answer 'd) No, I would not feel confident to apply an AED'. Following the presentation, the reverse occurs: 90%–95% of responses are 'a) Yes, without hesitation'.

Feedback
The feedback I receive is invariably along these lines:

> Thankyou, I understand what I need to do now and I am not frightened to do it.

> Thank you sincerely for a splendidly clear lecture on CPR and Defibrillation. You have removed the anxiety of not knowing enough about AED usage.

And more specifically:

> Thank you Anne for an intriguing, highly informative and relevant presentation. I have gained outstanding knowledge and understanding

of the defibrillator and its lifesaving capabilities for any critical situation I am in in the future. I now feel fully informed and confident about when I need to use the AED and how to use it efficiently and smoothly in a life crisis situation, which is fantastic empowering knowledge to have. *Alia Steglinski, Complete Form Fitness and Nutrition.*

Kew Neighbourhood Learning Centre received our own defibrillator in 2015 and undertook training with Anne Holland from Defib First. Coincidentally, we had just completed our annual CPR refresher training that week. The value of the AED training was extraordinary and timely. It reinforced the importance of those vital first 3 minutes and gave us all the confidence to use the AED without hesitation. We are so pleased to have a defibrillator here at the centre and cannot stress how important it is to have not only the AED but the quality training to support it. *Wendy Jones-Wade. House Relationships Coordinator, Kew Neighbourhood Learning Centre.*

Training all interested staff

Defib First has a 'How much do you know about defibrillators?' online survey. Responses from the survey support the premise that there is a significant lack of awareness in the general community about the availability and accessibility of AEDs. Of the respondents, approximately 90% agreed that everyone should know how to use an AED and that AEDs should be situated in workplaces and public spaces. Only 33%, however, actually knew that their own workplace, school or club had an AED. Of the 33% who knew that an AED was on the premises, 72% did not know where it was located.

Presenting to all interested staff in the workplace, not just the designated first aid officers, gets this vital message across – anyone can apply an AED and the more people who understand where it is located as well as how, why and when to apply it, the greater the number of potential survivors.

In Chapter 4 'Industry adoption of AEDs' I referred to a workplace death in South Australia in 2012. The cardiac arrest victim's colleagues, who were trained in first aid, valiantly tried to save him with CPR but did not apply the available AED.

In other situations, the first aid-trained officers are not always present when a medical emergency arises. As an example, one of my sons was working during a pre-Christmas weekend at his multi-level city office. A number of other staff were also working after hours. There are two AEDs in the building and my son asked his colleagues: If I (or someone else) had a cardiac arrest right now, would any of you know what to do or where to find an AED or why an AED would be needed? None of his colleagues knew how to treat a cardiac arrest or what an AED was, let alone that there were two in the building and where they were located.

As previously discussed, research suggests that it is crucial that staff also receive ongoing retraining and refresher courses to ensure they retain the knowledge, skills and most importantly the confidence required to use AEDs.

Choosing a training provider

When choosing a first aid provider for formal first aid training, cost should not be the criterion for selection.

Qualifications and experience
All professional first aid training providers in Australia must have a minimum qualification of TAE40110 – Certificate IV Training and Assessment, must be partnered with a registered training organisation (RTO) and ideally they will also be nurses, paramedics, health or rescue professionals who have the practical skills and medical background to be able to teach correct technique.

Up-to-date equipment
It is not helpful if the learning environment involves AED training devices that are outdated and sometimes quite antiquated. Too many training organisations use AED training devices that do not represent the current models which trainees are likely to encounter in a real-life rescue situation. I was horrified on one occasion in 2014 to witness a CPR course in which the participants were required to plug a very outdated trainer AED into an electrical power source and insert wires into the unit before applying the pads to the manikin 'victim'. The training device bore

absolutely no resemblance to a modern AED. Using such antiquated equipment instils yet another false fear in the rescuer. Can you imagine thinking that you could be faced with a cardiac arrest in the street and would have to find a power point before an AED could be applied to the victim? It is simply not the reality – AEDs have their own battery power and do not require connection to a power grid.

Maintaining AEDs

Even more alarming is the incidence of AEDs that have not been maintained over the years, and on the occasion that a life hangs in the balance, the unit is found to be non-operational. As described in Chapter 10 'How AEDs save lives', an inoperable AED at a tennis club in 2013 would have had catastrophic consequences if rescuers had not been able to access another unit installed in a neighbouring sports club. The managers of the sports club were not unduly concerned that the rescuers ran in and grabbed the AED off the wall. Obviously, it was urgently needed to save a life.

It never ceases to amuse me how clubs and businesses worry about keeping the AED secure and preventing unauthorised access to it, rather than worrying about the risks and delays associated with making the AED too difficult to retrieve. It is reassuring, though, that most people change their views very quickly when this is explained. It also goes without saying that AEDs should be well maintained in accordance with the individual manufacturer's specifications.[77]

Monitoring and servicing

It is equally important when providing training that participants understand that AEDs should be monitored and serviced in the same way that fire extinguishers are maintained. This is a requirement that needs to be regulated. All too often, when an AED is needed in a time-critical emergency, it has sat unnoticed for years and is found to be non-operational because it hasn't been maintained or consumables such as pads and batteries have expired and have not been replaced. Regular monitoring is vital and just plain common sense, but until there is a change in regulations, care of the AED is voluntary.

To encourage organisations to be vigilant, Defib First provides a monitoring protocol to every organisation where AED training is delivered so the units are regularly checked and are maintained in working order. Clubs and voluntary associations are also advised to include monitoring and maintenance of the AED as an item in the agenda for their annual general meeting so that the awareness is passed from one committee to the next and the unit is not forgotten.

Education is the key to a successful outcome

It is imperative that more AEDs be widely available, accessible and monitored. It is even more important that ordinary people are educated to have no fear or hesitation in applying them because the only definitive first aid treatment for a sudden cardiac arrest is early CPR and early defibrillation. Rescue is time critical – the sooner a victim is defibrillated the greater their chance of survival, both short term and long term. Neurological deficits (brain damage) and post-recovery complications are also dramatically reduced. The more people who take responsibility and learn how to become urban lifesavers, the fewer unnecessary deaths will result. There is the potential to save thousands of lives.

Part Four

BUSTING
THE MYTHS ABOUT
CARDIAC ARREST AND
DEFIBRILLATION

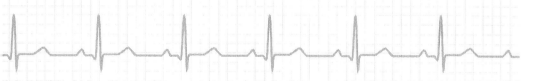

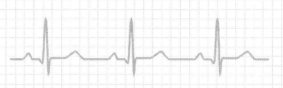

CHAPTER 13

MYTH 1 – SUDDEN CARDIAC ARREST IS A HEART ATTACK

*'Whether you believe you can do a thing or
believe you can't, you are right.'*

HENRY FORD

This book addresses seven myths about sudden cardiac arrest. The first and most common myth is that a sudden cardiac arrest (SCA) is a heart attack and therefore only happens to people who are unfit, overweight, older (predominantly male) with unhealthy lifestyles. The belief that SCA is a heart attack leads to the dangerous assumption that bystanders can do nothing because only doctors can treat a heart attack or it is not possible to save someone who 'drops dead' from a heart attack.

This belief that a SCA is a heart attack is ingrained in the community and the media, with the result that the two terms are used interchangeably. In the previously mentioned Defib First survey of public knowledge about SCA and defibrillation, over 75% of respondents believed that a cardiac arrest and a heart attack were one and the same. It is also quite common to hear the term 'massive' heart attack when someone suffers a cardiac arrest. The media perpetuates the myth by routinely reporting cardiac arrests as heart attacks.

Of even greater concern are medical, health and first aid-related sites that also refer to the same definition. In 2014, a large first aid training company was advocating, online, the importance of people learning about public access defibrillation (PAD) to treat 'heart attacks'. After it was requested that they amend their website to accurately refer to treating cardiac arrest not heart attack, to their credit, the text was changed.

The truth is SCA and heart attack are not the same condition – they are two separate events (although a heart attack can trigger a cardiac arrest as happened to my husband, Paul). Until the distinction is clearly made and understood, there will continue to be confusion on this critically important factor and therefore unnecessary deaths due to delay or, worse, inaction. Understanding the difference between SCA and heart attack will save lives.

As explained in Chapter 6 'What is sudden cardiac arrest?', a SCA is triggered by a malfunction of the heart's electrical system which causes the heart (*cardiac*) muscle to unexpectedly stop (*arrest*) beating. By contrast, a heart attack occurs when an artery supplying blood to the heart muscle becomes blocked.

A SCA is the end condition or terminal event of something else that has triggered it. Although a SCA most frequently occurs as a result of a heart attack (particularly in the early stages), there are many other causes of cardiac arrest that affect all age groups and both genders. Some of these causes are arrhythmias (abnormal heartbeats), drowning, asthma, fumes, smoke, choking, anaphylaxis, injury/trauma, blood loss, drug overdose, stroke, genetic disorders and electrocution.

What is a heart attack?

The medical term for a heart attack is acute myocardial infarction (AMI). *Myo* refers to muscle, *cardial* to heart, and *infarction* to tissue death (necrosis), which occurs when part of the heart muscle is starved of oxygen.

A heart attack occurs when a coronary artery (blood vessel that supplies blood to the heart muscle) suddenly becomes narrowed or blocked by plaque or a clot. The blockage prevents that section of the heart muscle from receiving its vital blood supply. This typically (but not always) causes chest pain and if the blockage is not cleared quickly the affected part of the heart muscle begins to die. The longer treatment is delayed, the greater the damage to the heart.

Every heart attack is very serious; however, heart attacks can be medically categorised as *mild* through to *severe* depending on the extent of the blockage and whether more than one artery is affected (there are multiple coronary arteries that supply blood to the heart muscle). The term 'massive' can be misinterpreted and misleading because a person can have a severe or 'massive' heart attack but still not have a cardiac arrest. Conversely, it is possible to have a mild heart attack but also go into cardiac arrest.

Heart attack victims frequently remain conscious and experience symptoms such as chest discomfort or pain and other identifiable signs and symptoms such as pressure, heaviness or tightness in one or more parts of the upper body including chest, neck, jaw, arm(s), shoulder(s) or back; nausea; shortness of breath; dizziness or a cold sweat; all of which can vary in severity.[78] Sometimes symptoms of restricted blood flow can also appear more slowly and persist as discomfort (a feeling like indigestion) for hours, days or weeks before the heart attack occurs. Symptoms can be brought on by excitement or exercise but sometimes there are no precipitating factors.

Heart disease is the number one cause of death in Australia and kills almost as many women (49%) as men (51%).[79] However, women usually present with different symptoms to men, which can disguise the true nature of the complaint. Women may experience symptoms such as shortness of breath, dizziness, nausea, back pain or just unexplained tiredness and fatigue. Women are more likely to call an ambulance for their husbands than for themselves. They often think that their warning signs are a less life-threatening condition such as indigestion and so they don't promptly call emergency medical services (EMS). In Australia, call Triple Zero (000).[80]

Many people have a heart attack without having a cardiac arrest, meaning their heart does not necessarily stop beating. However, it is true that a person having a heart attack is at very high risk of going into cardiac arrest because the heart muscle becomes irritable due to the reduced blood flow, and this can make it start beating erratically. An individual with a suspected heart attack still needs urgent medical attention. The importance of summoning immediate emergency medical aid cannot be over-emphasised. The person needs prompt treatment to limit the damage to their heart and to reduce the risk of SCA.

Heart attack or sudden cardiac arrest?

In summary, a heart attack occurs when blood flow to part of the heart muscle is blocked, while SCA occurs when the electrical control of the heart malfunctions and the heart suddenly stops beating without warning. It is possible to survive a heart attack but it is not possible to survive a cardiac arrest without defibrillation.

Heart attack	Sudden cardiac arrest
Plumbing problem (of circulation)	Electrical problem (of beating)
Awake (conscious)	Not awake (unconscious)
Breathing	Not breathing or not breathing normally
Responsive	Not responsive
Heart is still beating	Heart is not beating

Table 1. Comparison of heart attack and sudden cardiac arrest

What to do when a heart attack is suspected

A heart attack occurs every ten minutes in Australia. Over 50% of deaths from heart attack occur before the victim reaches hospital. Almost 25% of people who die from a heart attack die within one hour of their first warning sign.[81]

Someone who is having a heart attack cannot survive if the electrical system that controls the beating of their heart also malfunctions and they go into cardiac arrest. For those who do go into SCA, the only outcome for them is death unless they are treated immediately with cardiopulmonary resuscitation (CPR) and defibrillation.

No-one experiencing symptoms of a heart attack should ever drive themselves or allow others to drive them to hospital, nor should they go to their local doctor or wait till the symptoms subside. Always call EMS first without delay because of the high risk of a SCA.

A heart attack that progresses to sudden cardiac arrest

As soon as a heart attack is suspected, bystanders should phone for help, then bring the nearest available AED to the scene as a precaution. If the victim does go on to suffer a SCA while waiting for paramedics to arrive, then the AED can be used without delay to maximise the victim's chance of survival.

CASE STUDY: Heart attack progressing to cardiac arrest

A heart attack victim suffered a cardiac arrest while waiting for an ambulance, during an episode of Bondi Rescue, a reality TV show filmed at Sydney's famous Bondi Beach.

A 54-year-old man came out of the water in a distressed state. He had the classic signs and symptoms of a heart attack – severe chest pain, shortness of breath, sweaty and clammy skin and poor skin colour. He was lying on the sand and the lifeguards, having already phoned Triple Zero (000) for an ambulance, sent for the AED.

It is extremely likely that someone suffering a heart attack will go into cardiac arrest, so the lifeguards made the correct decision to put the AED electrode pads on the victim, even though he was still conscious and communicating with them.

The lifesavers knew that the AED would record the victim's heart rhythms which would be helpful for doctors who would later manage his condition in hospital. More importantly, with the pads already on the man's chest, if he went into cardiac arrest the AED would detect the lethal rhythm and deliver a shock without delay to defibrillate his heartbeat back to a normal rhythm.

At first, while the victim was conscious and therefore had a normal heartbeat, the AED did not deliver a shock, but just after the paramedics arrived he did in fact lose consciousness and go into cardiac arrest. The AED did its job and defibrillated him, while also recording all of the changes in his heart rhythm for later analysis.

The smart thinking of the Bondi lifeguards resulted in rapid defibrillation which saved his life.

If I was placed in the same situation and was dealing with someone who was conscious and presenting with a probable heart attack, I would also put the AED pads onto them. The AED will not deliver a shock if it is not required; however, it still detects and records the heart rhythms, which is very useful information for doctors. In the worst-case scenario, it would automatically advise and deliver a life-saving shock, if needed. If the patient did not require defibrillation, there would be a cost to replace the electrode pads which are disposable and for single use only. This is a small price to pay for peace of mind.

This episode (Season 9, Episode 9, Part 1) can be viewed on the official Bondi Rescue YouTube channel at: https://www.youtube.com/watch?v=CcqfI9jRbSE.

Why this myth needs to be busted

This myth is dangerous for the victim because it gives the rescuer a false belief that there is nothing they can do except wait for medical help to arrive, when in fact the opposite is true.

There are many causes of SCA and the precise cause can usually only be determined by medical tests in hospital. It is very important therefore to understand the distinction between SCA and heart attack. Too frequently, when someone collapses and stops breathing it is assumed that the casualty has suffered a heart attack, and bystanders are too fearful to take action because they believe that only paramedics, doctors and nurses can treat a heart attack or worse, the victim is beyond saving. The former part is true but the latter is not. A victim of heart attack does need urgent medical treatment from qualified personnel. However, that is of little consequence if the heart attack victim also suffers a SCA and does not receive immediate resuscitation on the spot.

Without treatment for the cardiac arrest, the person is dead and will remain dead. If the patient can be revived and transported alive to hospital, doctors can then diagnose and treat the heart attack, improving the victim's chance of survival. Without defibrillation for the cardiac arrest, the victim's heart attack (or whatever caused the cardiac arrest) will be diagnosed on autopsy.

It is true that the rescuer cannot treat the heart attack but they can treat the cardiac arrest and when 'regular' people do nothing during a cardiac arrest, they lose valuable time. It is so important to remember that cardiac arrest is the one cause of death that a bystander rescuer can reverse and restore a victim to life, if they apply an AED promptly. Ideally, an AED needs to be applied within three to five minutes of the cardiac arrest and the longer the delay before defibrillation, the lower the victim's chance of survival.

The rescuer does not need to focus on the cause unless there is danger to them or others. SCA can affect anyone, of any age, anytime, anywhere. Some people (young and old) can have a SCA unrelated to a heart attack and without warning signs, so we all need to be prepared to know how to deal with it. The bystander rescuer's only priority is to provide immediate lifesaving treatment, because regardless of the cause of a cardiac arrest, the first aid response is the same: CPR and defibrillation.[82]

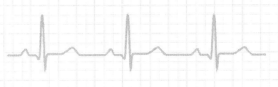

CHAPTER 14

MYTH 2 – RESCUERS CAN BE SUED FOR RENDERING FIRST AID

'Never doubt that a small group of thoughtful committed citizens can change the world. It's the only thing that ever has.'

MARGARET MEAD

Many people believe that they can be held liable and sued if they apply an automated external defibrillator (AED) and the outcome is not successful, in other words, if the patient does not survive.

Before addressing liability with respect to operating an AED or providing cardiopulmonary resuscitation (CPR), it is important to remember that an individual who is unconscious and is either not breathing or not breathing normally is in urgent need of resuscitation because they are in fact dead. It is therefore not possible to harm them any further. Any attempt to resuscitate the victim gives them some chance of survival and applying an AED gives them the greatest opportunity to recover.

It has been estimated that bystanders in the community render first aid treatment in less than 40% of cases due to fear of liability if they do something wrong. With that statistic applied to SCA, over 60% of cardiac arrest victims die unnecessarily without receiving any lifesaving help because rescuers (and workplaces) are fearful they could be held legally liable and potentially could be sued.

The truth is that the law, under 'Good Samaritan' legislation, protects anyone who renders first aid in good faith. In particular, no-one ever has or ever could be sued for attempting to resuscitate a victim of cardiac arrest by applying an AED because the victim is already dead.

What happens if we do nothing?

Without intervention, a victim of SCA has no chance of being revived and will certainly die. So in the case of an individual who is already deceased, it is almost nonsensical to worry about being held liable if the resuscitation outcome is not successful.

Good Samaritan legislation

AEDs are now so technologically advanced, reliable, safe and easy to use that most jurisdictions, including in the litigious United States, enshrine the use of an AED in 'good faith' by any person under 'Good Samaritan' laws. Good Samaritan legislation means that a volunteer responder cannot be held civilly liable for harm to or the death of a victim by providing improper or inadequate care, given that the harm or death was not intentional and the responder was acting within the limits of their training and in good faith. AEDs cannot be used inappropriately and create little liability.

Key terms defined

Good faith
In 2003, Michael Eburn (Associate Professor, College of Law, Australian National University) wrote in the *Australian Journal of Emergency Management* that the approach taken by the US state of California was that 'to act in good faith' was to act with 'that state of mind denoting honesty of purpose, freedom from intention to defraud, and, generally speaking, means being faithful to one's duty or obligation'. Associate Professor Eburn also referenced Australian High Court Justice McTiernan, who when considering a statutory immunity that applied to the New South Wales fire brigades, said that the concept of 'good faith' referred to an act that was done 'without any indirect or improper motive'. It would appear that a person who is providing emergency assistance acts in good faith when their honest intention is to assist the person concerned.[83]

Good Samaritan

Dr Sara Bird, a medico-legal claims manager, defined a Good Samaritan as:

> a person (including a medical practitioner) who in good faith and without expectation of payment or reward comes to the aid of an injured person, or person at risk of injury, with assistance or advice. There is an ethical and professional obligation on medical practitioners to act as Good Samaritans. In New South Wales and the Australian Capital Territory there is also a legislative duty on medical practitioners to provide assistance on request. Outside of these locations, there is no legal duty to provide assistance on request, except in the Northern Territory, where unique legislation requires any person to provide assistance to another irrespective of their training.[84]

Emergency

Although the term *emergency* is not generally defined, the (Australian) Acts are clearly directed at medical emergencies. They are intended to apply to Good Samaritans who are providing first aid or medical care to a person and will not apply to people who are acting to preserve property. In medical terms, a major accident or illness that is life-threatening and requires urgent treatment is an emergency. Cardiac arrest certainly fits within this description.

United States and Canada

There are cases of Good Samaritans legislation in practice around the globe, with some laws now making special mention of AEDs. For example, in order to help reduce delays in lifesaving care, the US state of Ohio enacted a new law in 2014 (House Bill 247) that permits anyone to perform external defibrillation to resuscitate another person, and protects them from liability.[85]

In addition to Good Samaritan laws, Ontario, Canada, also has the Chase McEachern Act (Heart Defibrillator Civil Liability) 2007, which protects individuals from liability for damages that may occur from their use of an AED to save someone's life at the immediate scene of an emergency, unless damages are caused by gross negligence.[86]

Australia

Associate Professor Eburn noted in 2003 that Australian governments had undertaken major reforms in the law of negligence. Legislation was introduced to limit the liability of Good Samaritans and voluntary members of community organisations. It applies, significantly, in emergencies where bystanders at the scene of an emergency come forward to assist. The legislation also protects volunteer members of the emergency services who respond as part of their duties.[87]

The legislation implemented a number of recommendations of the *Review of the Law of Negligence* by a panel headed by Mr Justice Ipp (the Ipp Committee). There is, or has been, a widespread fear that anyone, and doctors and nurses in particular, face a great risk of being sued should they stop to render assistance in an emergency. This fear exists despite the fact that there are simply no cases of anyone being sued in these circumstances. The Ipp Committee reported that:

> The Panel is not aware, from its researches or from submissions received by it, of any Australian case in which a Good Samaritan (a person who gives assistance in an emergency) has been sued by a person claiming that the actions of the Good Samaritan were negligent. Nor are we aware of any insurance-related difficulties in this area.[88]

Australian states and territories

Legislation exists in all Australian states and territories protecting Good Samaritans from liability 'in any civil proceeding for anything done, or not done, by him or her in good faith in providing assistance, advice or care at the scene of the emergency or accident'. Emergency assistance is, by definition, limited to medical assistance or other assistance to protect life and safety, not property.

The purpose of Good Samaritan legislation is to encourage people, particularly health care professionals, to assist strangers in need without the fear of legal repercussions from an error in treatment.

The Queensland legislation is the oldest Good Samaritan Act in Australia but its operation is limited to doctors and nurses. The other states and territories legislation provide Good Samaritan protection for anyone who acts in good faith and without expectation of payment or other reward to assist a person who is apparently injured or at risk of being injured.

Some jurisdictions require that Good Samaritans act not just in good faith but also without recklessness when coming to the aid of another who is in need or apparently in need of emergency assistance. Some states also have exclusions from protection if the Good Samaritan is intoxicated or impaired by recreational drugs.

Most of the Acts also protect a medically qualified person who, without expectation of payment, gives advice via telephone or other telecommunications device about the emergency treatment of a person.

A list of state and territory Good Samaritan legislation in Australia can be found in Appendix C.

Protection for community organisations

New South Wales, Victoria, Queensland, Western Australia and South Australia have also introduced legislation to protect volunteer members of community organisations. For example, in New South Wales a volunteer does not incur any personal civil liability in respect of any act or omission done or made by the volunteer in good faith when doing community work organised by a community organisation, or as an office holder of a community organisation.[89]

Why this myth needs to be busted

The myth that rescuers could be legally liable or could be sued is widespread and terribly dangerous because fear stops so many people from doing anything to help a victim in a medical emergency or accident. In the case of cardiac arrest, this means too many people die – not because they were going to die anyway, but because no-one took any first aid action. Without intervention by bystanders, a victim of cardiac arrest will certainly die.

The clear message is that there is no Australian case in which anyone (including health professionals) has been sued for negligence when they have voluntarily rendered emergency care in good faith.[90]

In a March 2014 blog post, Associate Professor Eburn stated that a rescuer (in particular, a health professional) cannot be liable if a patient does not recover because 'liability could only begin to be an issue if you make the situation worse so that the person would actually have been better off if you had not turned up at all'.[91] It is not possible to make the situation worse for someone in cardiac arrest – any attempt at resuscitation is better than no attempt.

An AED cannot be used inappropriately as it can only shock someone with a lethal and shockable heart rhythm (VF or VT), so an AED cannot harm a healthy person. When an AED administers a shock, it is delivered to someone who is already clinically dead, so no further harm can be done.

If there is a question of liability, it may now very well apply to not having an AED available, especially in the workplace, given that all first aid-trained personnel must now be competent in the use of an AED. This raises the question of duty of care when staff are trained to provide a skill in a medical emergency but are not supplied with the equipment with which to perform that skill.

In summary, the fear of liability is unfounded because Good Samaritan legislation exists around the world to protect rescuers from the risk of litigation when they act in good faith in an emergency.

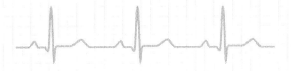

CHAPTER 15

MYTH 3 – AEDS CAN SHOCK SOMEONE WHO DOESN'T NEED TO BE SHOCKED

'At the end of the day, let there be no excuses,
no explanations, no regrets.'

STEVE MARABOLI

The popular belief is that an automated external defibrillator (AED) can:

- shock someone who doesn't need to be shocked
- shock the wrong person
- discharge a shock indiscriminately without warning.

These fears arise from folklore and misrepresented incidents on TV or in movies and even from slapstick comedy routines. These depictions may be contextually funny but have the potential to mislead people into forming incorrect assumptions and fears.

AEDs in popular culture

There is an episode of *Mr Bean* in which a man collapses at a bus stop, and in typical Bean fashion, the ensuing parody creates a farcical comedy of errors. The character Mr Bean pokes and prods the man for signs of life, then gives him 'CPR' which involves Mr Bean using his foot to perform compressions and giving mouth-to-mouth resuscitation by blowing through a rolled-up magazine. Eventually Mr Bean uses car battery jumper leads to first revive the victim and then to electrocute him when he regains consciousness.

While it is intended to be entertainment, the fallout may be very serious. Such exaggerated images can instil fear into the psyche of people who would then be reluctant to deal with a real-life situation. Their hesitancy to act could then result in the victim's death because no-one did anything to help.

This *Mr Bean* scenario is impossible in real life, yet it is so commonly referenced in pop culture that it creates yet another myth that people believe to be true. It leads people to worry that if they use an AED they will shock and injure themselves or someone else.

Unfounded fears

All of the fears associated with this myth are unfounded. The truth is modern AED technology is computerised, sophisticated, reliable and safe. It is just not possible to shock the wrong person or to shock someone who does not need to be shocked.

Layperson first aid rescuers consistently worry that the resuscitation will not have a successful outcome. For example, laypersons worry that the victim will die, or the AED will not work correctly and will discharge a shock without warning, or that they, the rescuers, could do something wrong. However, the AED pads must first be applied to the body of the victim, then the AED must analyse the heart rhythm and specifically detect a lethal shockable heart rhythm before it will advise that a shock is required, charge the energy and then deliver a shock. Therefore, an AED cannot be used inappropriately.

Importance of early defibrillation

Electrical defibrillation of a shockable rhythm detected by an AED is well established as the only effective first aid treatment for cardiac arrest. Basic cardiopulmonary resuscitation (CPR) life support will help to maintain blood circulation to the brain and heart muscle which prolongs a shockable rhythm but it is not a definitive treatment. The scientific evidence which supports early defibrillation is overwhelming. Defibrillation is the best chance of survival for a victim of SCA, if it is provided within the first few minutes.

Not everyone can be saved because there are many underlying causes of cardiac arrest. However, survival rates can be as high as 75%–85% if defibrillation is delivered promptly, compared with survival rates of less than 5% without early defibrillation. The figures speak for themselves and the importance of taking immediate action cannot be overstated. The delay from collapse to delivery of the first shock is the single most important determinant of survival. The chances of successful defibrillation decline at a rate of 9%–10% with each minute that defibrillation is delayed.

Resuscitation councils worldwide strongly recommend a policy of applying a defibrillator on victims of SCA with minimal delay.

Real-life examples

AEDs can be operated by virtually anyone and have been designed to be used by rescuers with little or no first aid experience. AEDs guide the rescuers through the defibrillation procedure with clear, audible and easy-to-understand instructions. AEDs cannot and will not shock a person who does not require it.

The excellent 2014 video clip from the Australian reality TV series *Bondi Rescue* (described in Chapter 13 'Myth 1 – Sudden cardiac arrest is a heart attack') demonstrates that an AED does not shock indiscriminately and only delivers a shock when required. The episode, recorded at Sydney's Bondi Beach, shows a 54-year-old man who came out of the water suffering symptoms of a heart attack. While waiting for paramedics, the lifeguards decided to apply the AED. Ordinarily, an AED would only be applied if the casualty was unconscious, was not responding and not breathing. In this instance, however, it was reasonable to assume that the casualty may go into cardiac arrest. Applying the AED was absolutely the correct decision to make.

As expected, after analysing the man's heart rhythm while he was conscious, the AED did not advise a shock because it had detected a normal heart rhythm. He did, however, go into cardiac arrest and stop breathing a short time later. The AED promptly recognised that his heart was in a fatal but shockable rhythm and defibrillated him. He survived his heart attack and the cardiac arrest.[91]

CASE STUDY: Training video with live 'victim' as a model

Last year I filmed a training video demonstrating the application of an AED in a simulated cardiac arrest scenario. The 'victim' was one of my sons, Xavier, who 'collapsed' on cue in the gym and the AED was applied to his chest. Of course, after analysing his heart rhythm, the AED detected a normal rhythm and did not advise a shock. For the remainder of the video clip, an AED training simulator was connected and used to complete the video of a 'shock' being delivered. My son was very much alive and well throughout the segment. An AED simply will not defibrillate someone who does not require it and it is not possible to accidentally shock the wrong person.

Time and time again, I visit premises for training to find that the AED has not even been taken out of the delivery box because staff members are too afraid to touch it. It is just as common to visit premises where an AED has been unpacked but not assembled (some models are delivered with the battery installed whereas some others require the battery pack to be inserted into the unit).

As mentioned in Chapter 12 'Why are education and training so important?', on one occasion I was presenting at a community sporting club in Melbourne (name withheld to protect the embarrassed) and the AED had been mounted on display in its wall bracket for a couple of months but the battery had not been inserted because the members did not know what to do. Had someone had a sudden cardiac arrest, the AED would have been inoperable, and in the panic and confusion it's unlikely anyone would remember where the battery had been placed (which happened to be in another room).

How can we be sure AEDs only shock when necessary?

An AED is a programmed electronic device that only delivers an electric shock to victims of cardiac arrest when the heart rhythm is one that is likely to respond to a shock. The AED must follow a sequence of coded instructions before arriving at its one purpose, that is, to deliver or not deliver a lifesaving dose of electrical energy after detecting heartbeats or rhythms and determining whether those rhythms are shockable or not.

Simplicity of operation is a key feature of AEDs – the steps and controls are kept to a minimum, time is not wasted and voice and visual prompts guide rescuers. Modern AEDs are suitable for use by both layperson rescuers and healthcare professionals.

It is important to repeat that, all too frequently, I hear from concerned would-be rescuers that they fear:

- the AED will fire off a shock before they are ready
- they will put the AED on someone and get it wrong because the victim didn't need it and the AED shocks them anyway and 'kills' them (remember the victim is dead so it is not possible to kill them.
- they will shock themselves instead of the casualty.

None of these scenarios can in fact happen because the electrode pads must first be placed on and adhered to the casualty's bare chest. Until the pads are in place, the AED will not proceed to the next step of detecting and analysing a heart rhythm, before advising any action. This means that the AED must first be applied to the victim's body so that it can find a heart rhythm and then determine whether it is a shockable, that is, life-threatening rhythm.

What happens once a shockable rhythm is detected?

If the AED determines that the victim has a shockable, life-threatening, abnormal heart rhythm, it will announce that a shock is advised and warn bystanders to stand clear. It will then charge and deliver the shock through the electrode pads on the casualty's chest. If the AED is unable to detect a shockable heart rhythm or if it detects a normal heart rhythm, it will state 'no shock advised' and will not discharge any electrical energy or 'shock'. It is therefore not possible for any of the three scenarios above to occur.

The electrical current from a defibrillator is programmed to travel between the pads/electrodes through the victim's chest wall to concentrate the shock on the heart muscle. Best safety practice is for all others to be clear and not in contact with the casualty. If someone is touching the casualty at the time of shock, the likelihood of being harmed is low. (The risk is potentially increased if the person who is touching the patient at the time of shock has an underlying cardiac abnormality themselves.)

The AED electrode pads are coated in a sticky, gel-like substance that provides a conduction medium or pathway for the current as well as adhesion to the skin for optimal concentrated delivery of the shock energy. Skin (without the conductive gel) is not a good conductor of electricity and when the shock is shared between the victim and the person touching them, it does not usually produce enough energy to cause harm to others. However, if someone is touching the victim then some of the electrical current could be dissipated and lost. This could leave less energy to reach the victim's heart, so the shock may be less effective for the person who actually needs it.

What if the victim is on a metal surface?

Metal provides a conduction pathway for electricity, however, the electrical current delivered by an AED is programmed to travel between the two electrode pads. It is highly unlikely the pads would be in contact with a metal surface (such as a stretcher) because an adult casualty would normally be lying on their back and the pads are placed on bare skin on the front of the body. If any part of the victim's bare skin is in contact with any metal, the likelihood of another person being affected by the shock is low. To be on the safe side, however, best practice is to place insulating material such as clothing or towels between the metal and the victim, which allows the AED to be used without risk. Defibrillation should certainly not be delayed if there is body contact with metal. Rescuers should instead stand well clear during delivery of the shock.

If the victim is wearing metal jewellery, it can be removed if easy to do so. The victim's wearing of metal jewellery, however, should not prevent or delay defibrillation because at worst a minor burn might result from the electrical current. The victim can recover from a burn.

For a small child, the AED pads can be applied to the front and back of the chest. In this case, it is necessary to ensure that the child is lying on a dry, non-metallic surface. The placement of electrode pads on young children is covered in more detail in Chapter 27 'Defibrillation'.

What if the victim is lying in water?

Similar principles apply to water which poses a danger when combined with electrical current. It is not safe or practicable for anyone to defibrillate a victim in a body of water such as a swimming pool or while still in the water at the beach. The rescuers must remove the casualty from the water before applying the AED pads.

If a victim is wet from droplets of rain or is dripping wet after being removed from a pool, this does not present a significant danger during defibrillation. As long as there is no direct contact between the rescuer and the victim when the shock is delivered, there is no direct pathway for the electricity to take that would cause the rescuer to experience a shock. All that is needed is common sense: rescuers should dry the victim's skin to achieve best adhesion of the electrodes and optimal discharge of the energy into the victim's chest, and take particular care to ensure that no-one is touching the victim when a shock is delivered.[93]

It is also not ideal for the casualty to be lying in a puddle of water with others standing around in the water when operating the AED, but this should not delay the defibrillation. Best practice is to move the casualty to a drier position. If this cannot be done quickly, placing a stretcher, blanket, towels, clothing, newspaper or cardboard, etc. under the patient to provide a drier surface is recommended. If this still cannot be achieved, rescuers should stand well clear of the patient during the moment of defibrillation and then resume normal resuscitation. Bystanders are also protected if they are wearing rubber- or plastic-soled shoes.

Typical AED instructions that safeguard the rescuer

To reassure the reader that AEDs cannot shock the wrong person, these are typical instructions given by an AED (in Australia). In this instance, the AED is a Cardiac Science G5 Powerheart which automatically commences operation when the lid is opened and issues the following voice prompts, which are also displayed visually in an LED screen:

- Stay calm – follow these instructions.
- Make sure 000 is called now.
- Begin by exposing patient's bare chest – remove or cut clothing if needed.
- When patient's chest is bare, remove white square package from lid of AED.
- Tear open package along dotted line and remove pads.
- Peel one of the white pads completely from the blue plastic; begin pulling from the tabbed corner.
- Placed one pad on bare upper [right] chest.
- Peel second pad and place on bare lower [left] chest as shown.
- Do not touch patient; analysing heart rhythm.
- Do not touch patient; analysing heart rhythm.
- Shock advised.
- Charging.
- Stand clear.
- Shock will be delivered in 3–2–1.
- Shock delivered.
- It is now safe to touch the patient.
- Start CPR – give 30 compressions then give 2 breaths. *A metronome rhythm will guide the rescuer through the compressions and rescue breaths. The cycle will repeat four more times for a total of 2 minutes.*
- *After 5 cycles or 2 minutes, the AED will instruct rescuers to* 'Stop CPR. Do not touch patient; analysing heart rhythm'; *The AED will re-analyse the victim's heart rhythm to determine if another shock is advised.*

The AED is programmed to detect whether the pads have been peeled and placed on the skin. If the AED detects that the first pad has not been peeled and placed on the skin, it will repeat the same instruction until the action is completed. That is, it will repeatedly say, 'Peel one of the white pads completely from the blue plastic; begin pulling from the tabbed corner'. When the AED detects that this step has been completed, it will proceed to the next step.

If the pads are not placed appropriately, the AED cannot detect a rhythm and therefore cannot deliver a shock. If, after 2 minutes of repeating the same instruction, the AED detects that the rescuer still has not peeled and placed the pads, it will automatically instruct the rescuer to start CPR. This is intended to avoid prolonged delays during which there is no CPR or defibrillation intervention, which would significantly reduce the victim's chances of survival.

Why this myth needs to be busted

The danger of this myth is that people who are fearful of accidentally shocking and harming themselves or someone else (who doesn't need to be shocked) may fail to use the AED on someone who actually does need it. The victim could die as a result.

The truth is that someone who is in cardiac arrest is already dead and if they are to survive it is critical to avoid any unnecessary delays. Potential rescuers need to rest assured that they will not shock someone who does not need to be shocked, shock the wrong person, or shock indiscriminately without warning when using an AED. The AED will only work if it detects a life-threatening heart rhythm and a lifesaving shock is required. If an AED is placed on someone and it detects a normal heart rhythm, it simply won't administer the shock – it will do no harm. If the AED advises 'no shock', the only cost is the expense to replace the electrode pads, which cannot be reused.

There are many varied AED models and designs but all are developed with reliability, ease of use and simplicity in mind. As long as the general principles behind AEDs are understood, it is possible to save someone's life without risk to others.

AEDs are designed so that they are safe for anyone to use, regardless of whether they have had first aid training. The instructions are clear, audible and easy to understand; the steps and controls are kept to a minimum; time is not wasted; and an AED cannot and will not shock a person who does not require it.

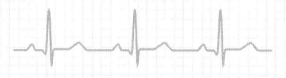

CHAPTER 16

MYTH 4 – AN AED COULD CAUSE FURTHER HARM OR INJURY TO THE VICTIM

'Our greatest weakness lies in giving up. The most certain way to succeed is always to try just one more time.'

THOMAS A EDISON

When I do automated external defibrillator (AED) presentations or provide formal first aid training, I often ask the attendees about their most common concerns in relation to applying an AED. For about 50% of attendees, fear of injuring the casualty is a major inhibitor. Unlike in the last myth, where laypersons worry about shocking someone who doesn't need it, in this instance they are fearful of doing more harm than good by administering a shock, such as breaking ribs or actually killing the casualty.

If it wasn't so serious, this myth would be funny because it is not possible to hurt or kill someone with an AED – anyone who is in cardiac arrest is already dead. Any assistance rendered to them can only be of benefit. Even if an AED was applied to someone who was not in cardiac arrest, it would do no harm because it would deliver a shock only if a lifesaving shock was required. More harm is done to the cardiac arrest victim by not rendering aid to them, because they remain deceased.

It is extremely common for laypersons to fear that they will cause an injury to someone who requires resuscitation. As a consequence, laypersons may be reluctant to start CPR or apply an AED. It is critical to remember that when faced with a sudden cardiac arrest, *any attempt at resuscitation is better than no attempt* and a rescuer can only help the victim, who will not have a chance without someone doing something.

After calling emergency services for someone who is unconscious, not responding and not breathing, the next step is to commence CPR, then apply an AED (if available) as soon as possible, ideally within three to five minutes. The AED will determine if a shock is required and will only deliver a lifesaving shock if necessary, so it can *do no harm*.

Why do people have this fear?

People who worry about causing an injury with an AED generally confuse that fear with the possibility of injuring the victim with compressions during CPR or actually causing electrocution with the shock from the AED.

It is true that when performing cardiopulmonary resuscitation (CPR) it is possible to break a victim's rib or cause bruising; however, these injuries are usually minor and will heal, provided the person has a chance of survival. Victims cannot recover from cardiac arrest without CPR and the application of an AED. They can, however, recover from a broken rib or some bruising. If they do not survive, broken ribs are irrelevant.

Rib fractures most frequently result from the rescuer using excessive force in compressions or placing the hands on the incorrect part of the chest. Broken ribs are not uncommon even in a controlled medical resuscitation environment. I have witnessed resuscitation efforts in hospitals where vigorous compressions have caused rib fractures but the patients survived and their fractures healed.

When faced with severe stress, such as a medical emergency, our bodies automatically release a surge of the adrenaline hormone. The release of hormones such as adrenaline and cortisol causes a stress response which speeds the heart rate, elevates the breathing rate, heightens awareness and anxiety, releases glucose into the bloodstream, increases blood flow to major muscle groups. All of these reactions give the body a burst of energy and strength. This is known as the 'fight/flight/freeze/feign' response.

This surge of hormones causes a normal human response, which is to start CPR with increased power and vigour. While this should not result in injury, it sometimes does. The adrenaline rush settles very quickly, however, and as we use our surge of energy, we settle into a rhythm and the force of compressions usually abates as fatigue increases. This response is normal and happens to everyone in the initial moments of an emergency. It is not something that should prevent us from acting.

Is it safe to perform CPR on someone who has a pulse?

There is also a belief that performing CPR on a person with a pulse (and therefore a normal heartbeat) can cause injury or even kill them.

Until 2006, resuscitation guidelines recommended that rescuers check whether the patient had a pulse (heartbeat) before checking the airway, sending for help and commencing CPR. The problem with that approach was that rescuers who were unfamiliar with feeling for pulses wasted critical time trying to find them before starting lifesaving treatment. Worse, if someone was in cardiac arrest, they would not have a pulse to find, so the delay in looking for something that is not there would make the victim's situation even more dire.

The reality is that someone who does not have a pulse cannot be breathing. Conversely, someone who has stopped breathing (for example, from drowning, choking or drug overdose) either does not have a pulse already or will not have a pulse for much longer if they do not resume breathing.

Changes to resuscitation guidelines 2006

The resuscitation guidelines were changed in 2006 to improve survival by making the assessment of the casualty easier and quicker for the rescuer to take appropriate action. Nowadays, unless a rescuer is medically trained, the recommendation is to check if the person is unconscious, unresponsive and not breathing or not breathing normally, rather than checking for pulses. If someone, who just moments earlier was behaving and breathing normally, suddenly collapses and is unresponsive, they are in trouble and need urgent medical assistance, regardless of the cause.

In a 2006 press release, the Australian Resuscitation Council (ARC) stated:

> There is considerable evidence that, when using the pulse check on someone who has suffered a cardiac arrest you have a 50:50 chance of correctly determining if a pulse is present or absent. In other words, it is just as useful as tossing a coin. The greatest risk is to patients who need CPR but don't get it because the rescuer falsely believes the pulse to be present. In this situation, the likelihood of survival falls dramatically. (Appendix D)

With respect to the belief that performing CPR on someone with a pulse (meaning, someone who is not in cardiac arrest) is harmful, the ARC further stated that:

> There is no evidence whatsoever that performing chest compressions on someone who has a pulse will cause harm, in fact the recommendation has been for decades that chest compressions should be performed in unconscious children where their pulse is slower than normal. The same is often the case for unconscious adults who have slow pulse rates. This has been done without harm and does not cause disturbances of heart rhythm. (Appendix D)

Furthermore, it is recommended practice to not stop compressions to check if the patient has resumed breathing immediately after delivery of a shock from an AED, but rather to continue chest compressions until the AED analyses the rhythm two minutes later. Even if the patient is showing signs of breathing, it is believed that these compressions are of greater benefit to the victim (as their heart resumes a normal rhythm) and the compressions are not considered to be harmful. The time wasted checking for signs of life can, in fact, compromise the victim's chance of survival if they are not yet breathing normally and are in urgent need of chest compressions to maintain blood circulation and perfusion. Even if the victim has a re-established pulse, the compressions are not harmful to them in this situation.

Why this myth needs to be busted

The danger of this myth is that fear of causing further harm to the victim can prevent rescuers from taking lifesaving action with an AED. The truth is you cannot kill or injure someone who is in cardiac arrest;

they are already dead so it is not possible to injure them any further. The AED will do no harm to someone who needs it – it can only save them. More harm is done to the victim by not rendering aid to them, because they have almost no chance of survival without early compressions and defibrillation.

While it is possible for a rescuer to bruise or fracture the victim's ribs when performing CPR, this should not stop the rescuer from performing compressions or using an AED. Remember, a casualty can recover from broken ribs. They cannot recover from sudden cardiac arrest without lifesaving intervention from bystanders, or more specifically, defibrillation.

The lesson is: doing nothing does more harm than administering CPR or using an AED because when you do nothing the person stays dead. Even if you are in doubt, just have a go and put the AED on – it will decide whether the victim needs a shock or not! You cannot hurt the victim with an AED and if they get a broken rib or bruising from CPR, it will heal, but only if the victim lives.

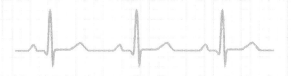

CHAPTER 17

MYTH 5 – PARAMEDICS WILL ARRIVE IN TIME

*'Change will not come if we wait for some other person
or some other time. We are the ones we've been waiting for.
We are the change that we seek.'*

BARACK OBAMA

When delivering first aid and defibrillation training, time and time again I encounter the general, misguided belief that an automated external defibrillator (AED) is not needed because all bystanders need to do is phone Triple Zero (000) and perform cardiopulmonary resuscitation (CPR) while waiting for paramedics to arrive with a defibrillator. Another misconception is that the hospital is just down the road and there will be enough time to get the casualty to the emergency department where a medical team will be waiting to swing into action and save the day. In other words, there is time to wait for someone else to take care of the situation.

These are Utopian ideals. However, survival from cardiac arrest just doesn't happen like that.

There is widespread misunderstanding that the role of bystanders is all about just doing CPR and that the time delay caused by waiting for paramedics, who are better qualified to use a defibrillator, is not really important. *Wrong!*

It is true that CPR is a critical stage of the chain of survival; however, an AED needs to be applied within the first three to five minutes for the greatest chance of survival and any delay in applying a defibrillator dramatically reduces the victim's likelihood of recovery. In Australia, ambulance response times are at times greater than 10 minutes and what many people don't realise or don't adequately understand is that getting to hospital takes time.

Why not just drive the victim to hospital?

Even if there is a hospital nearby, transporting a victim of sudden cardiac arrest (SCA) takes extraordinary effort and time. Someone who is in cardiac arrest is deceased; therefore, they are a dead weight. How much time and how many people would it take to move and carry a lifeless body (that has no blood and oxygen circulating to sustain them), get them into a vehicle and drive them to a hospital where they have to be removed from the vehicle and transferred into the emergency department before any resuscitation can be attempted?

To make the situation more impossible, while the victim is being driven to hospital someone may or may not be trying to perform CPR in a moving (speeding) vehicle, at unworkable angles and on inappropriate surfaces, to keep blood circulating long enough to get medical aid. The quality of the compressions would be ineffective and a waste of time. Trying to transport the victim to hospital just doesn't make sense and in fact gives the victim virtually no chance of survival. But people believe it is reasonable and doable, which just beggars belief.

The same argument, by the way, applies to someone who is possibly having a heart attack. As discussed in Chapter 13 'Myth 1 – Sudden cardiac arrest is a heart attack', the victim should not be driven to hospital or drive themselves because of the increased probability that they will go into cardiac arrest. An ambulance should always be called.

Why not just wait for an ambulance to arrive?

For those who think waiting for an ambulance during a cardiac arrest is the best option, even in the most ideal conditions an ambulance is not going to get to the casualty in less than five minutes, and depending on the circumstances, in Australia the response time is sometimes more than 10–15 minutes. Yes, good luck does prevail at times and paramedics may attend in less than 10 minutes but it is often just not possible to achieve that turnaround.

So many factors affect the availability of an ambulance – How far away is the nearest vehicle? Are they attending another job? Are emergency services stretched on this day or at this time? What are the traffic conditions? What are the weather conditions? What is the time of day? Is the area or building easily accessible? Where is the victim located? Is it easy to find the location? Is someone waiting to guide the paramedics to the scene? Is it a high-rise building? Are elevators available? How many floors of the building need to be covered? On arrival, is there a significant distance to cross before getting to the casualty, for example a golf course, parklands, beach areas? Are there any dangers or hindrances? There are so many variables, it is all but impossible to guarantee an ambulance will arrive with a defibrillator in time to give the casualty the best chance of survival.

Why should bystanders apply an AED?

Ambulance Victoria statistics for 2014 revealed that someone who is defibrillated by bystander witnesses is three times more likely to survive than someone who is not defibrillated until paramedics/medical aid arrive.[94]

In a recent Defib First online survey, over 90% of respondents were employed. Of that group, 33% knew that their workplace had an AED while 25% did not know whether their workplace had an AED or not. Of those who knew their workplace had an AED, 72% did not know where to find it, which would result in potentially fatal delays if they had to locate it quickly. Nearly 69% of respondents would not apply an AED if it was available, or would wait for someone else to do it, or didn't know what they would do!

Any delay in defibrillation dramatically reduces the likelihood that the victim will survive. For every minute that passes without defibrillation, the chance of survival drops by 9%–10%. Waiting for paramedics is simply not best practice, but if an AED is not available, the only option is to perform CPR while waiting for first responders or paramedics to arrive.

First 3-5 minutes are vital

An AED needs to be applied within the first three to five minutes after a cardiac arrest to give the victim the greatest chance of survival. As previously discussed, after 10 minutes the chance of recovery is very low.

The graph in Figure 7 also appears in 'Chapter 10 AEDs save lives'. It is repeated here because it is relevant to the context of this chapter. The graph depicts how a cardiac arrest would progress if there was no treatment or intervention, that is, no CPR and no defibrillation. In the early stages of cardiac arrest, although there is uncontrolled electrical activity with ventricular fibrillation (VF) and no effective circulation of blood, at least electrical energy is still being detected and recorded. In those first five minutes, it is highly likely that a shock from an AED would reverse the abnormal VF rhythm back to a normal heartbeat.

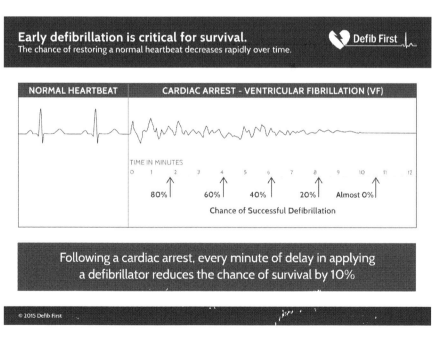

Figure 7. The chance of survival is greatest if an AED
is applied in the first five minutes

As the minutes pass without treatment, however, the tracing or recording of the electrical activity starts to get weaker until around the 8–10 minute mark, when electrical activity just tapers off and fades away to nothing. When there is no longer any electrical activity being recorded, the heart is in flat-line or cardiac standstill. At this point a defibrillator will not work because it cannot detect an abnormal rhythm; in other words, there is no electrical energy left in the heart, so there is no longer any fibrillation for the AED to terminate. Flat-line results from heart muscle cells dying and they cannot regenerate. The probability of recovery at this point is almost hopeless.

Best practice – MCG and Shrine of Remembrance

It is critical that CPR is performed to maintain a temporary circulation of blood, but rapid response with defibrillation is the key to survival. Excellent examples of best practice are the Melbourne Cricket Ground (MCG) and the Shrine of Remembrance in Melbourne which jointly have one of the highest (if not the highest) rates of cardiac arrest survival in the world (86%). There are AEDs placed at regular intervals around the facilities; there are teams of first responders who are trained and confident in applying defibrillators, and they don't waste time.

Minimising brain damage in survivors

Every minute of delay reduces the victim's chance of survival and dramatically increases the likelihood of complications with neurological (brain) damage and a compromised quality of life if they do survive.

A report in the American Heart Association (AHA) journal *Circulation*, 18 November 2014, concluded that, during a seven-year study period (2006–12) in The Netherlands, there was an increase in rates of survival after out-of-hospital cardiac arrest associated with increased AED use by witnesses at the scene of the arrest, along with improved neurological outcome (brain function). Survival increased at each stage of the resuscitation process, but the strongest trend was found in the 'prehospital' phase, that is, the treatment the casualty received at the scene before they arrived at hospital.

The proportion of surviving patients that had a favourable neurological outcome at discharge from hospital remained consistently high throughout the study period (89.9% in 2006 to 95.1% in 2012). Rates of AED use almost tripled during the study period (from 21.4% in 2006 to 59.3% in 2012), which reduced the time taken from placing a call to emergency medical services (EMS) to defibrillator connection. This increase in the use of AEDs statistically explains the increase in survival rate. The AHA recommended continuous efforts to improve resuscitation care, with strong emphasis on introducing or extending AED programs, involving both dispatched (EMS) AEDs and onsite (public access) AEDs.[95]

Survival rates with early defibrillation

The data collected by the AHA supports the2014 Victorian Ambulance Cardiac Arrest Registry (VACAR) report in Australia. The VACAR report revealed that victims of OHCA who received early defibrillation by bystanders were three times more likely to survive than OHCA victims who had to wait for EMS to arrive with a defibrillator.[96]

In the United States, the trend is similar. About 326,200 people experienced OHCA in 2011 (in 2014, the reported incidence varied between 350,000 and 424,000). Of those first treated by EMS in 2011, 10.6% survived. However, of the bystander-witnessed cases in which victims had a shockable heart rhythm and were treated effectively with an AED, 31.4% survived.[97]

Bobby V Khan, MD, PhD, director of Atlanta Vascular Research Foundation, who serves as board chair of the Sudden Cardiac Arrest Foundation said:

> The AHA report findings indicate that earlier intervention in cases of sudden cardiac arrest increases the chances of survival and a better quality of life. We must continue to emphasize the importance of doing whatever is possible to prevent sudden cardiac arrest – and we must continue to educate the public about what to do if they witness a sudden cardiac emergency.[98]

Why this myth needs to be busted

The myth that you can wait for paramedics when an AED is readily available, or can even transport a victim to a nearby hospital, is so very dangerous because precious time is lost either waiting for help that may not arrive in time, or worse, delivering a person to hospital in a condition from which they cannot be recovered because of the delay.

The lesson to be learned in busting this myth is every minute matters; time is critical – don't waste it. Delay costs lives and 'waiting for someone else' can be fatal.

Although the message is repetitive, early defibrillation is essential. Any delay in defibrillation dramatically reduces the likelihood that the victim will survive.

It is important to always remember that all is not lost if an AED is not on hand. It should never be assumed that the victim cannot survive with CPR only while waiting for paramedics. There are good news stories such as the rescue at Montara Wines, described in Chapter 10 'How AEDs save lives'. The reality is, however, that it is rare to have successful outcomes when first defibrillation is delayed.

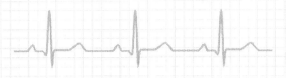

CHAPTER 18

MYTH 6 – ONLY QUALIFIED PROFESSIONALS CAN USE AN AED

*'Sometimes it's the people that no one imagines anything of,
that do the things that no one imagines.'*

THE IMITATION GAME

A common public perception is that only medical professionals, or at the very least first aid-trained personnel, are qualified to apply an automated external defibrillator (AED).

From another perspective, the bystander doesn't know what to do or how to use an AED so they do nothing and hope that someone more knowledgeable will come along.

It is understandable that layperson rescuers worry about things not working out well, or the AED not working, or that they could do something wrong and harm the victim or be sued; however, the International Liaison Committee on Resuscitation (ILCOR) – Consensus on Science and Treatment Recommendations made the following statement in 2010:

> An AED can be used safely and effectively without previous training. Therefore, the use of an AED should not be restricted to trained rescuers. However, training should be encouraged to help improve the time to shock delivery and correct pad placement.[99]

In the United States, the state of Ohio has even enacted legislation in December 2014 to protect and make it lawful for anyone to perform external defibrillation to resuscitate another person, which will help reduce delays in lifesaving care. Ohio law previously allowed defibrillation to be performed only by those with training in AED and cardiopulmonary resuscitation (CPR). The new law allows anyone to use an AED, and recommends training, but does not require it.

Karen Cromacks, an American Red Cross CPR and defibrillation teacher in Cincinnati said:

> When someone is suffering from a cardiac emergency, every minute of delay decreases their chance of survival by 10 percent. If using an AED machine required training by law then, when someone collapsed in a public place, you would have to start looking for someone with a card. That could cause a delay.
>
> AED machines send a strong electric shock to a heart that is in fibrillation. They are present in most public buildings [United States] and are designed to be used by people with little to no medical experience. The person using the machine doesn't make the decision whether to shock the person. The machine makes that decision. All you have to do is get the unit, get it on to the person's chest, and let the machine read the electro activity of the heart and make the decision.[100]

In short, while training is recommended, it is by no means essential, which means anyone can save a life.

What would you do?

Picture this scenario – Defibrillators are located throughout all airports and can be found, for example, on the walls in transit lounges and the arrivals and departures halls.

Imagine for a moment that you are standing at the baggage carousel of an airport waiting for your luggage and the person next to you suddenly collapses. Anyone who collapses suddenly is in need of urgent first aid assistance. However, in this instance the victim is not breathing or is not breathing normally, and is unresponsive and unconscious – they are in serious trouble because they are dead.

What would you do? Would you even know where to look for an AED? Would you race over, grab it from the wall and apply it to the victim? Many people wouldn't because they 'don't know what to do' or they 'feel foolish in front of all those people' or they fear 'doing something wrong' or they 'assume someone "trained" will race to the rescue and save the day'.

In the previously mentioned AED survey conducted on the Defib First website, only 31% of respondents indicated they would apply an AED without hesitation; this means that nearly 70% of respondents would wait for someone else to take the initiative.

Why do people hesitate?

The reasons why people assume only qualified professionals can use an AED once again come from lack of understanding, urban myth, pop culture and old wives' tales. Some of these reasons link into other myths, such as fear of making a mistake and harming the victim further, fear of accidentally shocking the wrong person, and fear of being sued if the outcome is unsuccessful.

But another significant reason people are hesitant to take action and apply an AED is the mistaken belief that AEDs are complex, unpredictable machines that can only be operated by professionals who have been trained on how, when and why to use them.

An interesting and gratifying anecdote recounted at the 2015 Australian Resuscitation Council 'Spark of Life' conference in Melbourne, was that in all instances of cardiac arrest at Melbourne Airport, witnesses actually applied an AED before the arrival of first responder teams. Luckily for those who have a cardiac arrest at Melbourne Airport, their rescuers are among the 31% of the population who would apply an AED without hesitation!

AEDs are automated and safe

The airport anecdote supports the reality that anyone, regardless of their level of first aid training, can safely and effectively apply an AED to someone who is in cardiac arrest – it is best practice to be trained but you don't need specialised training or even a first aid certificate. The key to survival is immediate CPR, and most importantly, early defibrillation. An AED is intelligent and automated. It tells the rescuer what to do and will only deliver a shock if advised. After the rescuer has called for help, all they need to do is to remove clothing from the victim's chest, apply the electrode pads and let the AED do the rest. An AED is fail-safe and cannot be used inappropriately.

Anyone, even a child, can do it

The message is repetitive, I know, but can't be overstated. Modern AEDs are technologically advanced and are designed to be used by bystanders, regardless of training. AEDs are programmed to guide the user through every step of the process. Before a shock can be advised, the AED pads must detect and analyse a heart rhythm in the same way that an ECG machine detects and records the heart rhythm when we have an electrocardiogram.

If an AED detects that the victim has a shockable fatal heart rhythm, it advises a shock is required and delivers that shock. Some AEDS will discharge the shock automatically, while others are semi-automated and instruct the rescuer to press a flashing button to discharge the energy. In either event, the AED is in control of delivering the shock. Even if the button on a semi-automated AED was pressed accidentally, the device would not discharge any electrical energy if it was not necessary.

Some AEDs can also assess the quality of the chest compressions and give real-time feedback to the rescuer: whether they are providing good compressions or whether they should press harder or faster to improve the quality of the compressions. All brands of AED supplied by Defib First have these capabilities.

Typical AED instructions to guide rescuers

To set the reader's mind at rest, here is another example of the types of loud and explicit instructions issued by an AED (this time the semi-automated HeartSine Samaritan 500P model).

Remain calm, call for help, retrieve the AED (only if close by, otherwise send someone else to retrieve it) and commence CPR. Remove the AED from its carry case and press the green button to start the prompts.

Ensure all upper body undergarments have been removed, excess hair has been shaved from patient's chest, if necessary, and skin is dry.

AED prompts from HeartSine Samaritan 500P:

- Adult patient – call for medical assistance.
- Remove clothing from patient's chest to expose bare skin.
- Pull green tab to remove pads.
- Peel pads from liner.
- Apply pads to patient's bare chest as shown in picture.
- Press pads firmly to patient's bare skin.
- Assessing heart rhythm; do not touch the patient.
- Analysing; do not touch the patient.
- Stand clear of patient – shock advised.
- Press the orange shock button (flashing) now.
- Shock delivered.
- Begin CPR – it is safe to touch the patient.
- Place overlapping hands in middle of chest.
- Press directly down on the chest in time with metronome.
- Remain calm.

What if the rescuer doesn't follow the AED instructions?

The instructions issued by an AED are very clear and allow the rescuer enough time to perform each task. If the rescuer performs the steps faster than the AED instructions, the AED will automatically keep up and proceed to the next instruction. So the protocol is ideal for both untrained and trained rescuers.

The victim is not left in 'limbo' if an AED is opened but the rescuer does not or cannot follow the instructions. If the rescuer has not followed instructions for two minutes, then the AED will automatically proceed to giving instructions for CPR.

For example, as discussed in Chapter 15, 'Myth 3 – An AED can shock someone who doesn't need it', when the lid of the Cardiac Science AED is opened, the AED automatically turns on. It issues the instruction to 'peel one of the white pads completely from the blue plastic; begin pulling from the tabbed corner', but if the AED detects that the rescuer has not completed the instruction, it will repeat the same instruction for 2 minutes. After 2 minutes and 10 seconds, if the AED cannot detect that the pads have been placed on the patient, it will automatically revert to instructing the rescuer to perform CPR. At the end of 2 minutes of CPR, the AED will return to the instructions to place pads, and once again, if it detects that there is non-compliance after 2 minutes, it will instruct the rescuer to recommence CPR.

This scenario is not a good outcome because the AED is not being deployed to analyse the victim's heart rhythm and therefore defibrillation (if needed) is being delayed. However, it is better to perform CPR than to just ignore the non-placement of the pads and allow the situation to progress without any CPR intervention, which would give the victim no chance of survival.

CASE STUDY: Police detain man for applying an AED

A bizarre example of this type of false perception occurred in Japan in 2011. A man was branded a 'pervert' when he stopped at a traffic collision and, after phoning for emergency services, began performing CPR on a female passenger who was unconscious.

An AED was obtained from a nearby store, and the Good Samaritan rescuer cut through the woman's clothing to expose her bare chest so that the adhesive electrode pads could be placed directly on her skin. (Clothing must be removed so the pads can be applied to bare skin. Underwiring in a bra can reduce the quality of compressions and also interfere with the delivery of the shock, so bras should be removed.)

The driver of the vehicle called police to report the stranger as a sexual molester and the police detained the rescuer for questioning.

There was a happy ending, though, because the woman survived and the stranger was thanked for his quick-thinking bravery and released by police. The lesson here is that if all parties concerned, including the police officers, had been better informed about using AEDs and had known that clothing must be removed for the application of an AED, there would not have been a waste of time nor trauma caused to the rescuer, who was acting appropriately.[101]

Why is community awareness so important?

Another fear which may prevent some potential rescuers from taking action is the worry that their attempts to help could be misunderstood, or even construed as harassment. Any rescuer, especially a stranger who acts quickly and applies an AED should be applauded for their role in giving the victim the greatest chance of survival.

Is training necessary?

Training in CPR and the use of an AED is recommended and desirable, and a rescuer is better prepared if they have had training. However, in a life-threatening situation such as a cardiac arrest, any delay can result in a poor outcome or unsuccessful revival. It is vital, therefore, to not waste time thinking about whether someone more qualified will come along. The victim has the best of chance of survival if immediate action is taken.

The AED will advise the rescuer to administer CPR; obviously it is far more preferable and helpful if the rescuer knows how to perform CPR effectively, but remember – *any attempt at resuscitation is better than no attempt.* So if the only action the rescuer takes is to apply the AED pads, at least the casualty has an opportunity to be defibrillated and a normal rhythm may be restored.

Further information on first aid training is contained in Chapter 12 'Why are education and training so important?'

Why this myth needs to be busted

The danger of this myth is that people either do not do anything when they witness someone collapse or they wait too long for someone else to take action. And, of course, this compromises the victim's chance of survival.

Under normal circumstances, there is a high likelihood that designated first aid responders will be on the scene quickly to take over. Airports, railway stations, sports arenas and other places where people gather in large numbers usually have AEDs and first responder teams ready to act.

But consider for a moment if there is a delay or no first responder readily available. What then? Who helps the victim? The risk is that if everyone assumes that someone else will do it, the victim can be surrounded by scores, even hundreds of people and none of them will do anything to assist the victim who then has no chance of recovery.

AEDs are designed to be used by either trained first responders or untrained laypersons. AEDs should be located in areas that are clearly visible, accessible and are not exposed to extreme temperatures. Their locations should also be clearly signed and they should be maintained according to the manufacturers' specifications so that they are always in rescue-ready mode.[102]

On the Defib First website (www.defibfirst.com.au) there is a free resuscitation chart and checklist download which can be printed and displayed prominently near the AED to assist rescuers with the most efficient procedure during a cardiac arrest.

The lesson is that sudden cardiac arrest is the one cause of death that bystanders can safely and effectively reverse by applying an AED, before emergency medical services arrive.

Anyone can be an urban lifesaver, so just apply the AED and let it work its magic.

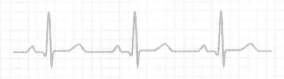

MYTH 7 – AN AED IN THE WORKPLACE INCREASES LIABILITY

'It always seems impossible until it is done.'

NELSON MANDELA

Does your workplace have an automated external defibrillator (AED)? The answer is: probably not.

Employers are frequently reluctant to install AEDs in the workplace. The most common concerns are that corporate liability risks for business would increase and management could be held liable and even sued if an AED was used inappropriately; if the victim did not survive; or if the wrong person was shocked. The common perception is that the business could be blamed for providing a dangerous piece of equipment that people were not adequately trained to use.

Many employers also resist installing an AED because they fear that their business would be sending a message to employees that the workplace is unsafe or stressful and likely to cause heart attacks. Therefore (as the next step in this thinking goes), the only reason an employer would have an AED on standby is because a heart attack is probably going to occur.

Frequently, the installation of an AED in the workplace or community space is actively resisted and opposed because people perceive that AEDs are unnecessary equipment, are expensive to purchase and costly to maintain.

It never ceases to astound me how much fear and misunderstanding exists in the community, and particularly in the workplace, about the application of AEDs in saving lives. These fears span a range of industries, including commercial, educational, sporting and voluntary organisations.

Regardless of the type of business or workplace, the common myths around AEDs prevail – that rescuers and/or employers can be sued; that an AED could shock the wrong person or cause further harm to the victim; that rescuers can wait for paramedics to arrive; or that specialised training is needed to operate an AED.

As has now been explained in busting the earlier myths, rescuers are protected by 'Good Samaritan' legislation; they cannot shock the wrong person with an AED or cause further harm to a victim; there is not enough time to wait for paramedics; and anyone can legally use an AED with or without training.

Education and increased public awareness are the only ways to address these fears. Once the fears are dispelled, the idea that an AED could increase an employer's liability becomes nonsensical.

The truth about workplace issues and resistance to AEDs

Liability

Firstly, having an AED on the premises does not increase an employer's liability. The reality is that, following 2013-2014 changes to first aid training requirements in Australia, the employer may in fact be more liable for *not* having an AED available and accessible.

The simple truth is there is no liability associated with having a defibrillator on site. Good Samaritan laws exist in Australia (and overseas) (as discussed in Chapter 14 'Myth 2 – Rescuers can be sued for rendering first aid') and no-one has been sued or held liable in Australia for providing first aid in good faith. This includes applying a defibrillator to someone in cardiac arrest. Repeating yet again, it is not possible to do any further harm or damage to a victim of sudden cardiac arrest (SCA) because they are already dead and any attempt to help them can only be of benefit. Not shocking the victim will ensure they remain dead! The victim's only hope of survival is time-critical intervention. Without cardiopulmonary resuscitation (CPR) and defibrillation, the victim cannot survive. Waiting for emergency medical services to arrive in order to provide defibrillation significantly reduces the victim's likelihood of survival.

Using an AED presents no personal liability because rescuers are protected by Good Samaritan laws and the reality is that an AED simply cannot be used inappropriately (Myths 2 and 3), but management still worries about increased liability from having an AED on site.

All teachers must have annual CPR training (which now includes competency in the use of an AED), and yet I have attended numerous schools to provide AED training only to find that staff members have not even opened the box containing the defibrillator. Either the staff did not know what to do with the AED or they were too frightened or unsure about touching it and wanted to wait until the trainer was present before unpacking it. It is surprising how many times this reluctance has occurred in schools, however, it does not pertain only to schools.

In one retail trading precinct in Melbourne (a prominent shopping strip, another name withheld to protect the embarrassed), an AED had been provided but was not available for public use for over twelve months because not one of the traders was willing to accept 'liability' for housing it. Eventually, the local independent supermarket agreed to provide a home for the AED. When I presented the much-promoted and long overdue training session for people who were wary of the AED, only one trader and the coordinator attended! These attitudes are representative of many businesses.

In September 2008, the Australian Resuscitation Council was provoked into releasing the following statement to counter erroneous media reports about the costs and liability associated with AEDs.

AUSTRALIAN RESUSCITATION COUNCIL

CHAIRMAN:
Assoc. Professor I G Jacobs BAppSc, DipEd, PhD, RN, FRCNA, FACAP
DEPUTY CHAIRMAN:
Dr P Morley MB BS, FRACP, FANZCA, FJFICM

SPONSORED BY
Royal Australasian College of Surgeons
Australian and New Zealand College
of Anaesthetists

PRESS RELEASE

Defibrillators in Public Places

During the past week newspaper reports have appeared that raises concern as to the placement of Automated External Defibrillators in public places, in this case railway stations in Sydney. In these articles it is stated that these defibrillators are complex devices to use, CitiRail staff may be held liable and questioning the cost.

The Australian Resuscitation Council (ARC) – Australia's peak body on issues relating to resuscitation – refutes the claims made in these articles. The provision of defibrillators in public places - a concept internationally known as Public Access Defibrillation - is now widespread in many places throughout the world including the United Kingdom, Europe, USA and in every State or Territory in Australia. These devices are easy to use and are now regarded as part of basic CPR training.

Evidence from a number of studies has clearly shown a greater chance of survival from cardiac arrest in places where defibrillators are publically available. Places where defibrillators have been located include airports, casinos, football stadiums, shopping centres and work locations. Have a closer look when next you are at an airport or shopping centre!!

The ARC unequivocally supports public access defibrillation and would congratulate RailCorp in undertaking this important public health initiative.

Associate Professor Ian Jacobs
Chairman

12 September 2008

Queries: Associate Professor Ian Jacobs   Mobile 0418916261

Australian Resuscitation Council Inc.
C/- Royal Australasian College of Surgeons
College of Surgeons' Gardens, Spring Street, Melbourne 3000
Telephone +61 3 9249 1214   Facsimile +61 3 9249 1216
e-mail: ARC@surgeons.org

In the United States, one of the most litigious countries in the world, AEDs are now so easy and safe to use that most states include the 'good faith' use of an AED by any person under Good Samaritan laws. Good faith protection means that a volunteer responder (trained or untrained) cannot be held civilly liable for the harm to or death of a victim by providing improper or inadequate care, given that the harm or death was not intentional and the responder was acting within the limits of their training and in good faith. (Good Samaritan legislation is covered in Chapter 14 'Myth 2 – Rescuers can be sued for rendering first aid'.

As mentioned in Chapter 18 'Myth 6 – Only qualified professionals can use an AED', in December 2014 the US state of Ohio enacted House Bill 247, permitting any person to use an AED to resuscitate another person, even if they have no training in how to use an AED. The law, which had previously provided immunity from civil lawsuits to those who use a defibrillator, now extends that immunity to anyone who owns an AED.

Dayton, Ohio, Fire Chief Jeffrey Payne said he hopes the law will encourage members of the public to take action in a crisis situation:

> We don't want people to think that they'll hurt someone by trying to use an AED machine. As long as they follow the instructions, it's really an effective tool, and it's very user-friendly. We don't want anyone to fear litigation for trying to help their fellow person.[103]

Workplace stress

Myth 1 established that cardiac arrest and heart attack are not the same event. Although stress can predispose an individual to a cardiac event, there is no direct link to the workplace environment. Other physiological factors would coexist with stress to produce a heart attack.

A cardiac arrest has no warning signs and can strike anyone, of any age, anywhere, anytime. Seventy-five per cent of cardiac arrests occur outside of a hospital, so an AED is the most vital component of emergency first aid equipment. CPR prolongs life until defibrillation, which is the only effective first aid treatment for cardiac arrest. Although a cardiac arrest can result from a heart attack, they are not the same condition. SCA can have many different causes.

Having an AED on the premises does not mean a workplace is stressful and more likely to produce heart attacks. The concept of an AED giving a business a bad reputation is unfounded and illogical. On the contrary, having an AED on the premises actually enhances safety and reduces liability and risk in the workplace. If employers are concerned that this myth is true, it is further evidence that more education is required to correct the misinformation.

Workplaces are required to have fire extinguishers and evacuation plans but that doesn't mean staff and customers assume that those environments are more likely to have a fire. Fire extinguishers are a form of insurance and are one of the reasons why fatalities caused by fire are so low. Apart from preventing deaths, without fire extinguishers, regular staff training and drills and maintenance of the equipment, workplaces would be in breach of occupational health and safety (OH&S) or workplace health and safety (WHS) laws. An AED should have the same status.

The same OH&S requirements pertain to the shipping, cruising, boating and aquatic activities industries as well as the airline industry. Life rafts, life vests, buoyancy devices and electronic position indicating radio beacons (EPIRB) are standard equipment and in some situations, compulsory equipment, in the event that a rescue at sea or in other bodies of water is needed. Safety protective equipment promotes preservation of life in the event of an incident involving water.

The number of deaths caused by SCA however far exceeds (by many thousands), the number caused by drowning which was approximately 452 (excluding bathtub deaths) in 2013 in Australia.[104] SCA occurs 73 times more frequently than drowning. In industries where water is a health and safety risk, individual life vests and other buoyancy devices must be provided to prevent drowning. Only one AED would need to be available in each location to treat cardiac arrest and yet this critical piece of lifesaving equipment is not compulsory.

Expenditure

AEDs in Australia are relatively inexpensive (generally between A$2,000–A$3,000). They last for many years, come with seven to 10-year warranties and have long-life batteries. Amortised over a 10-year period, an average AED investment would cost less than $300 per annum.

Even with the inclusion of replacement costs of consumables for the AED, for just $300 a year, a workplace could save a life (not to mention also save on the costs of time lost due to injury and lack of productivity, replacement and training of personnel, termination and sick-leave payouts, and potential liability and compliance). An AED, like a fire extinguisher and a first aid kit, is insurance for a business and is a justifiable expense.

Implication of changes to first aid training regulations

In Australia, workplaces with 10 or more employees (the number varies around the country) are required to provide first aid kits and have designated staff trained in providing first aid. CPR is an essential first aid skill when responding to a SCA because it buys the victim time, but on its own, CPR does not restore a normal heart rhythm.

As previously mentioned, from July 2014, it has been regulated in Australian first aid training that participants must also be assessed as competent in operating an AED. However it is not compulsory to actually provide the AED in the workplace first aid kit. In other words, employers are training staff to perform a lifesaving skill but they are not required to provide the necessary equipment to implement that skill.

A valid argument exists that defibrillators should be an essential inclusion in first aid kits in the workplace to reduce the risk of an unsuccessful outcome, that is, the death of an employee, volunteer or visitor on the premises. The question could legitimately be asked: rather than being liable for having an AED on site, is the employer more liable for not providing the equipment they have trained their staff to operate, and which could actually save a life during a SCA?

So what could the implications be for businesses if the outcome is unsuccessful (i.e. someone dies) because staff lacked the availability of equipment they needed to perform the lifesaving duties for which they had been trained? Could the business owner be held civilly liable for the victim's death because an AED wasn't available?

The changes to training requirements are detailed in Chapter 1 'A case for providing AEDs in the workplace' and in Appendix B.

Workplace survival – a good news story

As described in Chapter 4 'Industry adoption of AEDs', Samantha Jobe was a fit, healthy, athletic 32-year-old new mother when she suffered a SCA at the Crossfit121 gym in Cheltenham, Melbourne, in 2014 in front of her husband and two-month-old baby daughter. If BASF, the company next door, had not installed an AED only weeks earlier, and had not told the surrounding businesses where it was located, it is unlikely Sam would have survived.

When Sam collapsed, her fitness trainers, Chris and Maria Hogan and Tara Smith, phoned Triple Zero (000) and started CPR. Maria, despite being seven months pregnant, ran next door to retrieve the AED. With the help of BASF workers, the AED was applied to Sam and it automatically delivered a lifesaving shock.

The following day, Ambulance Victoria paramedics attended the gym and downloaded the record of the event from the AED's memory to give doctors a better understanding of what had happened and what type of rhythms Sam's heart was in during the cardiac arrest. The cause of Sam's cardiac arrest was not a heart attack. A definitive diagnosis has still not been made, although an arrhythmia is the prime suspect. She now has an implantable cardioverter-defibrillator (ICD or internal defibrillator) surgically inserted in her chest and it has since saved her life a second time. ICDs are so sophisticated that Sam can transmit the recordings from her ICD to her cardiac clinic via a remote monitor at her home. She does not have to be taken directly to an emergency department unless she loses consciousness. Sam and her family are living proof that AEDs are effective and they represent the good news stories that can result, if only all workplaces were more responsive and proactive.

Sam believes that there should be legislation requiring AEDs to be located in all schools, sporting venues and clubs, gyms, and wherever people congregate. She is also convinced that she has recovered with no cognitive or memory deficits because her urban lifesaver rescuers started CPR so quickly. By performing rescue breaths as well as compressions, Sam's rescuers maintained air and oxygen flow into her lungs so it could be circulated to her vital organs.

A combination of the right equipment (an AED) and the right knowledge (where to find it and confidence to use it) means this is a workplace good news success story not a tragedy. Raising awareness is the key to getting the message across to all workplaces!

BASF Australia

The BASF story is a compelling example of why employers should not have any fear of or resistance to providing AEDs in the workplace. BASF has a very strong culture of safety and of caring about its employees. When BASF conducted a first aid training session at their Cheltenham site, they identified that the location of the nearest AED was a considerable distance away and decided to install a unit.

The defibrillator was purchased to enhance BASF's health and safety programs. Unlike a fire extinguisher, a defibrillator is not a mandatory piece of safety equipment, but both can save lives, so BASF's program went 'beyond compliance' to show commitment to its employees. The cost was considered immaterial, compared with the price of a life!

BASF is committed to a Responsible Care Management System. Once the AED was purchased, BASF promoted the program by advising all staff, creating flyers and, during the company's Global Safety Day, approaching immediate neighbours to advise them that the defibrillator would be available to them if they ever needed it. The AED was placed in a prominent position, right next to the front door of the premises, with appropriate signage.

In December 2014, Maria and Chris Hogan and Tara Smith from Crossfit121, with the two BASF workers, were nominated for Ambulance Victoria Community Hero awards and received their awards at Government House, Melbourne. The BASF site in Cheltenham was commended by Ambulance Victoria for 'outstanding efforts in purchasing a defibrillator and notifying neighbouring businesses of its availability in emergency situations.'

These health and safety endorsements must strip away any remnants of doubt regarding this myth.

The impact of BASF's corporate social responsibility and engagement with the community was very easy to measure – a human life was saved. BASF has helped raise the bar when it comes to workplace health and safety.

The Australian fitness industry

Maria Hogan, co-owner/trainer of Crossfit121, Cheltenham, is a passionate advocate of providing AEDs in gyms and fitness centres. Following Sam's successful resuscitation, there was significant media interest with interviews, news reports and articles.

In an interview for an industry related blog article, Maria made the point that an AED from another business saved Samantha's life and she emphasised how important it was for physical training studios, small and large gyms, and people who are trained in parks to have an AED available because these businesses are pushing high-risk clients, who may be overweight, unfit and not healthy, to their physical limits. Maria repeatedly referred to the importance of AEDs and the power that the fitness industry associations have to require members to provide an AED as part of accreditation, especially since AED competency is now compulsory in CPR training and all trainers must obtain annual accreditation of competency.

Maria was dismayed that the published blog did not reference her calls for changes to be made to fitness industry recommendations, especially since Samantha's physical condition and cardiac arrest didn't place her in the high-risk (overweight, unhealthy, unfit) demographic. In other words, SCA can happen to anyone and without an AED the outlook is not optimistic. Fitness Australia's 2014 Risk Management Manual says:

> There may be concerns from Fitness Facilities regarding the use of AEDs in the event the AED has a malfunction issue, or that training employees to operate AEDs might expose the operator and/or facility to liability, should the client not fully recover. However, in Australia, there are 'Good Samaritan-style' laws that recognise this concern and aim to protect rescuers who use AEDs from lawsuits.

Fitness Australia's risk management strategies recommend that all risks related to AED equipment can be managed and minimised by undertaking the following actions:

1. Discuss liability issues with your facility's legal adviser (and risk management committee). AED purchases should meet their approval and should be included in the facility's EAP.
2. Contact your insurance company to find out about potential coverage issues specific to your current insurance policy.
3. Maintain the AEDs in accordance with the manufacturer's specifications and the requirements of the *Work Health and Safety Act 2011* and *Managing Risks of Plant in the Workplace 2012*.
4. Establish and maintain a record keeping system of staff qualifications, competencies and training undertaken in respect to AED use.
5. Ensure accredited, appropriate training for safe use of AED equipment is provided to staff, with at least annual refresher training scheduled and access to re-certification made available.
6. Review the use of the AED(s) in your facility and ensure each incident requiring AED is documented.
7. Ensure the AED is well secured to minimise the risk of machine theft, but still allowing immediate access when required.
8. Create a system to provide post-incident support to the operator of the AED.[105]

Although regular physical activity clearly reduces a person's risk of acquiring cardiovascular disease, evidence suggests that in a small proportion of people heavy physical exertion may be a 'trigger' for an acute coronary event and subsequent cardiac arrest.

In the 2012 *Joint statement on early access to defibrillation*, the Australian Resuscitation Council, National Heart Foundation and St John Ambulance recommended that:

AEDs should be accessible in places considered high risk of a sudden cardiac arrest such as health and fitness centres, sporting clubs, other registered clubs (i.e. senior citizens), major events and across settings with employees, students, or clients with known risk of heart attack. Some jurisdictions are acknowledging the importance of early access to defibrillation in settings considered 'high-risk,' with the Western Australian Government considering legislation that would make the installation of AEDs into commercial fitness centres mandatory. (Appendix A)

Economic impact on business

Out-of-hospital cardiac arrest (OHCA) resulting in SCA is the foremost cause of death and the economic burden on the public health budget has been discussed in Chapter 3 'Roadblocks to providing AEDs in the workplace'. These unexpected deaths also clearly have an impact on productivity and flow on costs to industry because so many individuals are in their working years.

It is estimated that there are 33,000 cases of SCA in Australia each year, with the majority occurring out of hospital. Survival rates are still too low and the subsequent costs to business and government resources are high.

When avoidable deaths occur, in addition to the costs incurred by the employer, there are compensation payouts from insurance companies and superannuation funds. There are also resultant costs which affect the taxpayer purse such as supporting families that are left without a breadwinner. Then there are the medical costs of caring for a victim of cardiac arrest who may have survived but will never work again due to long-term medical complications, related to delays in emergency treatment.

SCA is eminently treatable in the workplace with prompt CPR and early access to defibrillation – the most vital link in the universally recognised 'chain of survival'. The time taken to defibrillation is a key predictor of survival. However, availability of a public access defibrillator is, unfortunately, the most frequently missing link in the chain. For a reasonable cost, employers can be industry leaders at the forefront of providing a safer workplace to prevent unnecessary deaths. At the same time, this modest 'insurance' investment can save businesses substantial costs in the longer term.

Corporate social responsibility – what can be done by industry?

Corporate social responsibility (CSR) encourages companies to have a positive impact (through their activities) on the environment, consumers, employees, communities, stakeholders and all other members of the public. Providing an AED lifesaving device would most definitely fit within the parameters of CSR.

All businesses are concerned with safety, governance, compliance, liability, care, lost time injury, reportable case injury and how to encourage employees to take ownership of safety, for example, regarding an AED as personal protective equipment (PPE). Some companies make safety a core value. There are also productivity, sick-leave management, duty of care, mental health and staff morale issues to consider.

As discussed in Chapter 5 'Summary of workplace concerns and obligations', workplaces are increasingly being identified as avenues for health promotion and health education for the workforce in Australia. Laypersons having access to and using AEDs for out-of-hospital cardiac arrest (OHCA) has gained increasing support but there is a long way to go before businesses are providing AEDs and making them more accessible when a SCA occurs.

When one considers how much money is spent by industry to protect data and property, a modest investment to protect life is not a significant burden on operational expenditure.

Why this myth needs to be busted

Workplaces can lead the way in providing a safer environment for all employees, clients and visitors on their premises. The seven myths about AEDs have been busted. There is no longer any reason why these lifesaving devices should not be integral components of first aid management in the workplace. Furthermore, following the changes in first aid training regulations, the time may be approaching when a workplace could be held civilly liable for *not* having an AED available.

The conclusion of the 2012 *Joint statement on early access to defibrillation* (see Appendix A) highlighted that early access to defibrillation is vital to improving outcomes from SCA. AEDs in the public domain (such as at major airports, shopping centres and sporting stadiums) have been shown to reduce time to defibrillation and save lives. Furthermore, first responder programs are effective in reducing time to defibrillation and provide a smooth transition to prehospital emergency medical services.

The 2014 VACAR evidence now supports that early defibrillation by bystanders triples the likelihood of survival.

St John Ambulance Australia, the Australian Resuscitation Council and the National Heart Foundation called upon the federal and state and territory governments to take the lead in developing and implementing early access defibrillation policy, ensuring the 30,000 plus Australians who suffer OHCA every year are given the best chance of survival (see Appendix A).

Like a lifesaving vest or a fire extinguisher, an AED is insurance. Hopefully it will never be needed but, if it is, an AED could save a life. The benefits of AEDs in the workplace are:

- optimising health, safety and wellbeing at low cost, A$2,000–A$3,000.
- improving staff morale and sense of security in a workplace that values safety
- potentially saving the lives of staff, customers and visitors
- reducing lost time injury and sick-leave payments
- saving costs by not losing an employee and having to train a replacement
- avoiding potential liability for not having a defibrillator in the first aid kit.

Keep in mind that not all victims of SCA die. Some will recover, but the time needed for recovery and the extent to which they resume normal life activities can be in direct proportion to the length of time before defibrillation takes place. Therefore, consider what it might cost industry and government and families if a staff member suffers a cardiac arrest and is off sick, or can only return to limited duties, or is unable to return to work at all.

Supermarkets are the obvious and most logical locations for the next step in the nationwide rollout of public access defibrillators because they are at the hub of every residential and retail community. They are open the longest hours, are highly visible and provide the greatest accessibility to an AED.

AEDs placed in supermarkets, high rise buildings, major retailers and commercial precincts would significantly enhance the chance of getting the AED to the victim quickly and optimise their chance of survival.

Ideally, following the example already set by Asda in the United Kingdom, supermarket and major retail chains around the world, starting with Australia, would install an AED in every store in the country.

Businesses could improve accessibility to AEDs by placing them on every floor or in every elevator of their multi storey buildings. Development and construction companies could lead the way to improving access to AEDs by making them standard inclusions in all elevators of future developments. Wherever there is a life vest or fire-fighting equipment, there should also be an AED.

What's impossible today, won't be tomorrow.

Part Five

DRSABCD

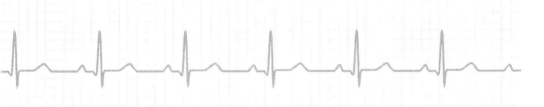

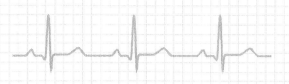

CHAPTER 20

EMERGENCY ACTION PLAN

'Step by step and the thing is done.'

CHARLES ATLAS

It takes a system to save a life. The DRSABCD medical emergency action plan (EAP) covers the seven steps to administering effective first aid during a sudden cardiac arrest (SCA) emergency. The chapters that follow will explain why these actions are recommended and why the EAP is so important for the chain of survival.

When confronted with fear, an emergency or a stressful situation, the body's automatic biological reaction is to release a surge of the hormone adrenaline to assist in the flight/fight/freeze/feign response.

Adrenaline increases the heart rate and respiratory (breathing) rate, increases agitation and anxiety and can contribute to confusion and a state of panic as the body is on high alert for immediate action.

Although it is beneficial that the body is prepared to take immediate action in an emergency, it can also be detrimental if the rescuer cannot think clearly or is agitated and confused.

For everyone confronted with the care and treatment of casualties, the EAP known as DRSABCD is a very useful tool to help the rescuer follow a sequence of seven steps related to **D**anger, patient **R**esponsiveness, **S**ending for help, clearing **A**irway, assessing **B**reathing, starting **C**ompressions and applying **D**efibrillation.

DRSABCD is the primary protocol (known as the primary action plan) for everyone involved in the care and treatment of casualties but it is also an essential aid in helping the rescuer to calm their nerves and think more clearly.

In the course of everyday life, most people see DRSABCD posters in their environment and their brains unconsciously change gear to 'ho-hum' mode. Generally, individuals believe they are familiar enough with the steps of DRSABCD and would know how to implement them in an emergency – *which is never going to happen to them anyway*!

In reality, without regular practice and familiarisation, once the adrenaline rush hits the nervous system, alarm and anxiety make it very difficult to remember clearly what to do and in what sequence to achieve a successful outcome. As a result, important steps can be overlooked, or followed incorrectly.

When a cardiac arrest is the medical emergency, implementing the chain of survival quickly and effectively can mean the difference between life and death for the victim.

Having DRSABCD signs on display in multiple locations provides quick and ready access to the emergency steps and a clear reference for the rescuer to follow, which helps to reassure the rescuer and also minimise time delays. It is a handy hint to carry a DRSABCD chart in the purse or wallet for speedy retrieval. A DRSABCD bookmark that can be folded into wallet size is an inclusion with this book.

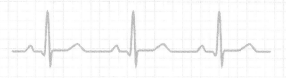

CHAPTER 21

DANGER – HAZARDS, RISKS, OBSTRUCTIONS, SAFETY ISSUES

'The wise does at once what the fool does at last.'

BALTASAR GRACIAN

Danger is the first contingency to consider in any emergency action plan (EAP), because although it may seem contradictory, you must always ensure your own safety as the rescuer first. If you are not safe, you are of no use to the casualty or anyone else and you can compromise a successful rescue. Putting yourself at risk in a dangerous situation may increase the number of casualties to manage.

For example, it is not uncommon to hear a report that a Good Samaritan died on a busy highway, after they stopped their vehicle to assist someone in distress. Without properly assessing the traffic dangers, they have left their vehicle and have been struck and killed by an oncoming vehicle or they have left their own car running and it has rolled and crushed them or someone else.

The second step is to assess the risk to and ensure the safety of the casualty and other bystanders in the vicinity by conducting a primary survey of the scene around you. Surveying the scene is important and can usually be completed quickly without compromising the rescue of the casualty.

Examples of danger/hazards/risks:

- electricity or power lines
- water and slippery surfaces
- fire, smoke, gases, fumes, chemicals

- traffic – both vehicular and pedestrian
- operating equipment
- individuals affected by drugs or alcohol or mental illness
- animals
- construction sites, unstable structures
- flammable materials, explosive risks.

Let's consider the scenario of someone mowing their lawn in a busy street with their loyal and large dog nearby. You are driving along the street and witness the person collapse on the side of the road. What are the dangers that need to be managed before you even assess the condition of the unconscious person? In this scenario, danger management could look something like this:

1. Ensure that you stop your car safely, park it securely out of harm's way and turn off the engine. Use hazards lights to alert other drivers.
2. Watch for other vehicles and signal to drivers to slow down and avoid the emergency.
3. Turn off the power to the lawnmower.
4. You may have to deal with an aggressive dog trying to protect its owner.
5. Ensure the casualty is not in further danger from roadside hazards and is not at risk of injury from other vehicles.
6. The person's family might happen upon the scene, become distressed or hysterical and require reassurance.
7. Passers-by might gather and create a hindrance which requires crowd management.

There could be many factors to consider, and most of the time the surroundings would be relatively easy to survey and control. However, it would be very stressful to be faced with any circumstance in which a person has stopped breathing and needs urgent attention, if the situation was dangerous and unmanageable. In that instance, there is little option other than to wait for the arrival of emergency services personnel who have the training and equipment to secure the scene.

Crowd management at the scene

The most common and troublesome 'danger' or obstacle in a rescue situation is not necessarily dangerous. It is usually other people (adults, children, adolescents) who can impede the rescue effort by being hysterical, obstructive, panic-stricken or overbearing. They may even faint. Hysteria and panic are very common behaviours in an emergency and in order to give the victim the best chance of recovery, it is extremely important that the scene be managed well.

This situation happened to me: an elderly gentleman, James (over 90 years old and pushing a walking frame) tried to cross a busy road between vehicles that had stopped for lights at an intersection 100 metres away. He made the mistake of crossing in front of a truck, which started moving when the lights turned green ahead. The driver was too high in the cab to see James, and as the truck rolled, it knocked him over. James was conscious and lying underneath the cabin of the truck between the front wheels. He was bleeding from superficial lacerations.

A doctor, who had stopped his car to help, and I ended up under the truck with James. He was on his side and breathing so we opted not to move him until emergency services arrived in case he had internal or spinal injuries. We focused on stabilising and reassuring him and managing his wounds. The major problem we had, however, was everyone else who thought they knew better. They were shouting instructions at poor James (who was in shock) and asking him questions such as his daughter's phone number! The doctor and I could not hear each other speak while we were trying to assess James's injuries. Eventually, I had to stick my head out from under the truck and 'request' that the onlookers keep quiet and back away.

Emergency procedure checklist

Having a rescue policy and procedure protocol or checklist in place is good forward planning. The most effective way of managing an emergency event is to give people things to do, using reassuring but clear, firm instructions:

- Encourage them to calm down, breathe slowly.
- Minimise conversation to the essential facts and duties.
- Designate a task for others to perform, such as
  - » phone EMS (000) and maintain communication with the emergency operator
  - » commence CPR
  - » retrieve the AED and first aid kit
  - » wait for paramedics to arrive and guide them to the scene
  - » manage bystanders especially those who hinder the situation
  - » direct traffic or set up perimeters
  - » reassure relatives or other distressed onlookers
- If unable to calm a distraught or obstructive onlooker, try to remove them from the scene.

To move or not to move the casualty

A casualty should be assessed in the position in which they are found, and rolled into the recovery position if they are unconscious and breathing normally. Unless their airway is compromised, it is not advisable to move an unconscious person, especially if the cause of their condition is not clear and movement may injure them further.

If, however, there is a hazard that cannot be secured, such as power lines, dangerous traffic, a body of water, a fire or poisonous fumes, there may be no choice and the casualty should be moved with care and with appropriate manual handling procedure while supporting the head and neck. If a lone rescuer has to move an adult casualty: gently roll them onto their back while supporting the head and neck and drag them by the ankles or wrists.

Ideally, moving a casualty should not be attempted until emergency services personnel arrive. They have the training and equipment necessary to protect themselves and the casualty but sometimes moving the casualty cannot be avoided.

In the case of sudden cardiac arrest (SCA), the casualty is already deceased and no further harm can be done to them. The casualty must be moved into a position suitable for cardiopulmonary resuscitation (CPR) and application of an automated external defibrillator (AED); otherwise they will not survive.

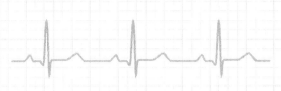

CHAPTER 22

RESPONSE

'Don't let what you cannot do interfere with what you can do.'

JOHN R WOODEN

After determining that there is no imminent danger, the next step is to assess the casualty for signs of responsiveness.

Someone who has gone into cardiac arrest is unconscious and will not respond to any verbal or tactile (touch) stimulus. They would give no response if you:

- asked them to open their eyes, move their limbs or poke out their tongue
- poked, prodded, nudged or shook them
- inflicted any painful stimuli such as pinching or rubbing their skin vigorously.

Aggressively shaking a casualty to gain a response is not usually necessary. Touching, gently shaking and talking loudly will awaken a sleeping person. A casualty that is unresponsive should be considered unconscious until proven otherwise. *Do not ever shake children and infants.* Shaking a baby or young child can jolt the brain around inside the skull, causing brain injury.

How to check for a response

Many first aid training providers recommend the 'talk and touch' method to check for a response, by asking some simple questions and giving some basic commands for the victim to follow.

Fainting vs. cardiac arrest

It is important to differentiate someone who is unconscious and not responsive in cardiac arrest from someone who has fainted. A fainting episode (also called syncope, pronounced 'sin-ko-pea', or a vaso-vagal attack) is a temporary loss of consciousness with a spontaneous recovery. It is a mild form of shock which occurs when there is a drop in blood pressure with temporary reduction in blood flow and, therefore, in oxygen supply to the brain. Fainting is frequently due to a drop in blood pressure and causes light-headedness, nausea/woozy feeling and a 'black out'. Someone who has fainted would appear pale but generally recovers or responds very quickly once they become horizontal. This is because the blood pressure rapidly stabilises when the casualty is lying flat and normal blood pressure restores adequate blood flow to the brain.

A casualty in cardiac arrest, however, will not respond regardless of which position they are in because the heart has stopped beating and therefore there is no effective blood pressure or circulation. The casualty's skin colour rapidly changes to dusky blue/purple tones, known as *cyanosis* (pronounced 'sigh-an-oh-sis').

I am not an advocate of the following method; however, it is frequently recommended so is worth discussing. COWS is a common acronym used to assist rescuers to remember what to do.

Can you hear me?
Open your eyes.
What is your name?
Squeeze my hand.

The reason I don't like COWS is because if someone is in cardiac arrest, they are incapable of responding. Waiting for the casualty to answer the questions or obey commands can waste critical time, especially if the casualty is making unusual noises, which can happen at the start of a cardiac arrest. The rescuer who hears these noises could be confused about whether the casualty is genuinely responding or not.

Someone who has suddenly collapsed and appears to be in an altered conscious state, but is not necessarily unconscious, may be affected by reduced oxygen flow to the brain (hypoxia) and may therefore be in a confused, incoherent, drowsy, semiconscious condition. In this case, the casualty's responses would be inappropriate, delayed or even absent.

In these circumstances, asking the casualty to answer questions and obey commands can take precious time that could otherwise be applied to resuscitation.

It is fine to ask these questions (COWS) once it is established that the person is breathing because then the rescuer is not dealing with a cardiac arrest emergency and can take time to assess the casualty's level of consciousness by questioning them and waiting for any responses.

When teaching, I always recommend that rescuers quickly assess response in this order:

1. Firmly prod the victim, calling out to them at the same time. It is fine to give instructions, such as 'open your eyes', provided there is no waste of time.
2. If no reaction, send for help immediately or instruct someone else to call emergency medical services (EMS).
3. Rapidly move on to assess the airway and breathing.
4. If the casualty is not breathing, commence cardiopulmonary resuscitation (CPR) immediately and apply AED if available.
5. If the casualty is breathing, then ask the questions (COWS) to assess conscious state.
6. If there is no response to questions and the casualty is unconscious but breathing, move them into the recovery position.

Some would say 'what does it matter?' because all of these actions can be achieved in a short period of time. This is true, but elapsed time in a cardiac arrest scenario is critical to survival and any time saved in the sequence can only help the victim. More specifically, rescuers are often unsure and slow when making this primary assessment so the time lost with unnecessary action can be significant.

Squeezing both hands

There is one other COWS rescue action that, in my opinion, is risky for the layperson (for two reasons) and that is asking the victim to squeeze your hand.

First, whenever an emergency occurs, bystanders are naturally anxious and can be hyper-energised or agitated. When asking the victim to squeeze their hand, an inexperienced rescuer can mistake their own firm or shaky hand grip as a reaction from the victim and may believe that the victim is responding when in fact they are not.

Second, if the victim has suffered a stroke (cerebrovascular accident (CVA)), there is the possibility that one side of the body could be paralysed (hemiplegia). If the rescuer only asks the victim to squeeze one hand, they may reach the wrong conclusion depending on whether or not they get a response of movement. The rescuer has possibly asked the casualty to squeeze with a hand that is paralysed.

In the medical world, when asking a patient to squeeze your hand to determine if they can respond, there are two rules:

1. Using both your hands, place two extended fingers (index and middle) into the palms of each of the casualty's hands between their thumb and forefinger. By using only the two fingers and not the full hand grip, the rescuer avoids misinterpreting their own grip movement for that of the patient.
2. Ask the patient to squeeze the (rescuer's) fingers with both of their hands at the same time, to assess that their grip strength is present and equal on both sides of the body. This method gives the rescuer more reliable information about the casualty's condition.

This is good practice for anyone assessing someone's condition by using any of the COWS steps.

Monitoring the casualty

If the casualty is able to respond to verbal stimuli by answering or appears to be conscious, do not move them unless there is potential danger or risk. Monitor their condition and try to establish what has happened to cause them to collapse. If necessary, send for help and reassess their conscious state regularly while waiting for emergency services to arrive. Now it is advisable to conduct a secondary survey to check for other injuries or bleeding. If, at any time, the casualty loses consciousness but is still breathing, place them in recovery position to protect their airway.

Assessing response from a stranger

It is possible to check a casualty's response by touching their shoulder and gently shaking them; however, it is not advisable to get too close to someone you do not know until satisfied that they are in fact unconscious. Unless you know the person, it is sometimes impossible to gauge if they are feigning for ill intent or are affected by alcohol or other drugs, or have a mental health condition. The rescuer's first priority is to avoid placing themselves in danger. Getting down close to a casualty can place the rescuer within grabbing range of the person's arms, if the 'casualty' does not respond as expected.

The best way to approach this assessment is to call out to the casualty for a verbal response and stand at their feet, away from their potentially grasping arms. The rescuer can use their foot to firmly (not violently) tap the casualty's foot. In this way, the rescuer can determine any response in a genuinely unconscious person but the rescuer remains in an upright position in case there is a need to back away quickly.

Why does 'send for help' come next in DRSABCD?

In past years, first aid rescuers were trained to check for airway, breathing and pulses (circulation), in that order, before phoning for an ambulance. The view now is that someone who was functioning and behaving normally one moment but who collapses suddenly, and is unconscious and non-responsive, is obviously in serious trouble and in need of urgent medical assistance. Immediate action is needed and the earlier emergency services are called and are on the way the better the outcome for everyone. So the next step is to send for help.

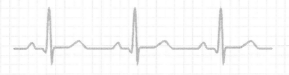

CHAPTER 23

SEND FOR HELP

*'Be strong enough to stand alone, smart enough to
know when you need help, brave enough to ask for it.'*

ZIAD K ABDELNOUR

Sending for help, or calling emergency medical services (EMS) for an ambulance, was moved up in the sequence of the emergency action plan (EAP) for a number of reasons. It was not uncommon for bystanders responding to an emergency to get flustered or distracted by rendering assistance to the victim and forget to actually call for help. This delay resulted in a loss of critical time and potentially compromised the rescue and likelihood of survival.

In addition, bystanders sometimes call the local doctor, hospital, family member or friend first, before phoning for an ambulance. These inappropriate calls cause delays and also significantly reduce the likelihood of survival.

Emergency dispatch is the anchor link in the chain of survival. Making 'send for help' a priority step in the plan reminds rescuers of the vital need to get medical aid on the way. Time is life and rapid dispatch of EMS, ideally in less than 60 seconds, significantly improves the victim's chance of a recovery.

Previously, it was recommended to check airway, breathing and circulation before calling for paramedics, but now it is recognised that sending for help earlier in the sequence gets emergency assistance on the way. Calling EMS also helps to support the rescuer because the EMS operators can offer information and instructions to assist the resuscitation and also monitor the progress of the incident.

It is important to send for help as early as possible by:

- shouting to alert nearby people
- sending someone to get or call for help
- using any phone available to alert the emergency medical service (EMS)by calling
  - » Triple Zero (000) in Australia
  - » 911 in North America
  - » 999 in Great Britain and parts of Europe
- asking others to find and bring an AED if available
- only leaving the casualty to get help when there is no other alternative.

Dealing with a medical emergency involving young children or infants

Special first aid consideration for young children or infants:

- If it is necessary to leave a child or infant in order to call for help, perform one minute of CPR first. In the absence of trauma or poisoning, young children and infants are more likely to have stopped breathing due to a respiratory problem; for example, drowning, suffocation or choking, and sometimes a short period of CPR can be enough to stimulate their breathing again.
- If the child or infant has any history of heart disease, call for help first without any delay.
- If there is only one rescuer, it is sometimes possible to carry a small child or baby to get help while performing CPR on the way – this is a very difficult decision to make and depends upon the location and circumstances.
- If there is more than one rescuer, one always starts CPR while someone else gets help.

Sending for help early is the first step in the chain of survival. There are a number of benefits from early recognition that help is needed and early access to assistance which give the casualty the greatest chance of survival:

1. Once a life-threatening situation has been identified as a Priority Code, the emergency operator will dispatch paramedics immediately, even while taking further details from the caller. This means that help is on the way at the earliest possible moment.
2. Unless there is a major disaster in the city or state where the call is being taken, the emergency operator will stay on the line with rescuers and advise and assist them in managing the casualty, especially in delivering CPR.
3. The operator can continue to gather information from the caller to be relayed to emergency services while they are on their way to the scene.

What to expect when making a Triple Zero (000) call in Australia

The Australian Medical Priority Dispatch System (MPDS) is a computer-aided dispatch (CAD) call-taking service focused on the chain of survival system of care which is only as strong as its weakest link. The call takers place great emphasis on rapid recognition of sudden cardiac arrest and immediate dispatch of EMS to minimise the response time which directly affects survival.

Initial questions
The questions asked by the Triple Zero (000) Telstra call centre operator will be:

1. Police, fire or ambulance?
2. Which state are you in?

Police, fire or ambulance?
The caller can specify which emergency service they require but the Telstra operator can also assist with this decision. Often, in a life-threatening emergency, more than one service will be dispatched. For example, it is not unusual for the fire brigade to be dispatched as well as an ambulance. Fire crews also carry defibrillators and can sometimes get to the casualty before or at the same time as paramedics.

Which state are you in?

When the Telstra operator asks 'which state are you in?', the operator is *not* asking how the caller is feeling emotionally (and yes, that question has been misinterpreted!) The question is intended to specify which state or territory the caller is located in. This is an important question.

If the emergency call comes from a fixed home phone or landline, the billing address of that phone is visible to the operator – and in the majority of cases, that's where the emergency services will be needed. But sometimes phone numbers are transferred to new addresses which may not yet be in the system or other technical issues may exist. So it is imperative that the Triple Zero (000) operator confirms the correct location for the emergency.

These days, most calls are made from a mobile phone and in that instance the Telstra operator will ask in which state the emergency is located. This is because a mobile phone number only shows the billing address, not a GPS location. The mobile phone billing address may not be the location where the emergency is taking place.

In the age of mobile media, the technology to accurately locate the caller via GPS coordinates is being developed but is not yet available. It is therefore critical for the operator to get accurate details starting with the state where the caller is located, so that the call can be transferred to the correct service.

Transferring your call

At this point, the Telstra call centre operator will transfer the caller to the appropriate emergency service in the relevant state and the emergency service operator will take over.

It is vital to not get frustrated with the questions asked. They are specifically framed for a variety of reasons, all of which are intended to result in the best response to the situation and in the shortest possible time.

Additional questions

Once a Triple Zero (000) operator identifies the location and that the caller is dealing with a Priority Code emergency (highest, life-threatening category), an ambulance will be routinely and quickly dispatched and on the road. The operator will ask additional questions to help gather as much information as possible. Answering these questions helps the operator to prioritise the emergency promptly and determine whether the casualty requires additional resources such as more ambulances, mobile intensive care ambulance (MICA) paramedic skills, fire brigade, police or other services.

Emergency services will be on the way and all other information gathered by the operator will be relayed in transit. It is important to stay calm and answer questions clearly and concisely. Some questions the emergency operator may ask include:

- The exact location of the emergency – Where is the nearest cross street or landmark?
- The direction of travel or the nearest exit or town if the caller is on a motorway or rural road.
- What is the phone number of the caller?
- What is the problem, what exactly happened?
- Is the person conscious (awake)?
- Is the person breathing?
- How old is the person?
- How many people are hurt?
- Are there any hazards or dangers?

It is crucial to stay on the line and not hang up. Follow the instructions offered by the emergency services operator, which will help the victim and the ambulance paramedics.[106]

An example of the efficiency and helpfulness of our EMS call takers occurred on the day that my husband Paul died. One of my sons, Xavier, found his Dad with 16 yr old Damien nearby. In the shock and hysteria that naturally followed my daughter, Bridgette, ran upstairs and rang 000 on her mobile phone. By this time, I was with Paul and would not allow my children in the room. The 000 operator asked to speak with me and, as Bridgette handed the mobile through the crack in the door, I accidentally disconnected the call with my thumb. I started to call back but, before I could hit '0' a second time, the operator had phoned me back. It was a first class response.

Emergency numbers

In Australia, the primary emergency call service number is Triple Zero (000), which can be dialled from any fixed phone, mobile phone or pay phone, and from certain Voice over Internet Protocol (VoIP) services. All of these calls to emergency numbers in Australia are free of charge. The call will be answered by one of two Telstra emergency dedicated call centres.

It is important to remember that in order to avoid potential confusion when using alphanumeric keypads, the pronunciation is 'Triple Zero' and not 'Triple Oh'. The letter 'Oh' on a keypad is number '6' and it is possible for people, including elderly persons, visitors to Australia, immigrants and those for whom English is a second language, to incorrectly dial '666' in an emergency.

Alternative emergency numbers

106 – Text Emergency Relay Service
For individuals who have a hearing or speech impairment, the Australian 106 Text Emergency Relay Service is available 24 hours a day, 365 days a year. Calls made using the 106 service are toll-free and are given priority over other National Relay Service (NRS) calls.

NRS '106' operators will communicate with the caller via a telephone typewriter (TTY) service or textphone. To indicate which emergency service is needed, the caller types 'PPP' (police), 'FFF' (fire brigade) or 'AAA' (ambulance). Operators will relay information to the appropriate emergency services operator and will also stay on the line.

The 106 service can only be dialled from a TTY and cannot be used by an ordinary phone, text message (SMS) on a mobile phone, or internet relay. As a TTY is connected to a fixed phone line, the emergency service operator can determine where the caller is located, although the caller will still be asked to confirm the address.

112 – International standard emergency number for mobiles

Triple Zero (000) is Australia's primary and recommended telephone number to call for assistance in life-threatening or time-critical emergency situations. Dialling 112 directs you to the same Triple Zero call service and does not give your call priority over Triple Zero. There is no advantage to dialling 112 over Triple Zero. It is *not* true that 112 is the only number that will work on a mobile phone.

The number 112 is an international standard emergency number which can only be dialled on a digital mobile phone. It is accepted as a secondary international emergency number in some parts of the world, including Australia, and can be dialled in areas of GSM (Global System for Mobile Communications) network coverage with the call automatically translated to that country's emergency number. Dialling 112 does not require a SIM card or PIN to make the call; however, telecommunications coverage must be within range of a transmission tower or satellite (via any carrier) for the call to proceed.

Dialling 112 from a fixed-line telephone in Australia (including payphones) *will not* connect you to the Triple Zero (000) emergency call service because 112 is only available from digital mobile phones. It is best practice in Australia to always dial Triple Zero (000).

Voice over Internet Protocol (VoIP)

Voice over Internet Protocol (VoIP) is a technology that allows telephone calls to be made over broadband internet connections. It is important to check with the VoIP provider if emergency call service is required because not all VoIP providers provide access to emergency calls.

911 – United States and Canada

Nine-one-one (911) is the emergency telephone number used in the United States and Canada but due to exposure to American media, movies and TV programs, it has become ingrained in the memory of many Australians who automatically dial it in an emergency.

Triple Zero (000) *not* 911 should always be used in an emergency in Australia.

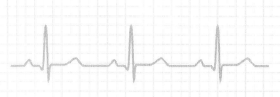

CHAPTER 24

AIRWAY

'Start where you are. Use what you have. Do what you can.'

ARTHUR ASHE

When someone's breathing has stopped or they are making strange noises and not breathing normally, it is critical to ensure that they have a clear airway. Checking inside the casualty's mouth and rolling them over to clear the airway, if is it obstructed, needs to be done quickly as time should not be wasted before starting chest compressions.

It is vitally important to ensure that the casualty's airway is clear for two reasons:

1. If the casualty has collapsed for a reason other than cardiac arrest and has not actually stopped breathing, clearing the airway will assist them to resume breathing normally. If the airway is not cleared, the blockage could prevent air getting to the lungs and therefore prevent breathing, which will lead to a cardiac arrest.
2. If the casualty is in cardiac arrest, they have stopped breathing, so getting air into their lungs with rescue breaths is vital for their survival. Even if the rescuer chooses not to give mouth-to-mouth rescue breaths, clearing the airway can allow air to move passively in and out of the lungs while compressions are being performed (more about that later).

There is an unpleasant reality of a casualty in cardiac arrest: it is likely that they have stomach contents, saliva/mucous secretions or even blood in their mouth or throat which can obstruct the airway into the lungs. Once someone is unconscious, every muscle in the body relaxes and the opening between the stomach and the food pipe or gullet (*oesophagus –*

pronounced 'ih-sof-uh-gus') also becomes relaxed or flaccid. The result is the possible escape (regurgitation) of stomach contents back up into the throat, mouth and air passages. This is potentially dangerous. There is a risk that the air passages could become blocked or the acidic stomach contents could flow back down (aspirate) into the lungs which would cause serious damage to the membranes lining the lungs.

Other secretions such as saliva, mucous or blood can pool when someone is unconscious and these fluids need to be drained or wiped away to prevent backflow or aspiration. Blood is sometimes present if the casualty accidentally injures themselves or bites their tongue or inside the mouth when they collapse. Water is present in cases of drowning. Foreign bodies may also be present, for example, if a child chokes on a small object or food lodges in a victim's airway.

If the airway (windpipe or *trachea* – pronounced 'track-ee-uh') is obstructed or blocked for whatever reason, the movement of air and oxygen into the lungs is therefore compromised or restricted.

Checking the airway

When checking whether the airway is clear, it is important to avoid wasting precious time and moving the casualty unnecessarily, so do not roll the casualty over straight away. At first, it is important that the rescuer only looks inside the mouth, by gently moving the chin slightly away – just enough to be able to see inside the mouth.

When there is an obstruction in the mouth and throat from secretions, water, blood, stomach contents or a foreign body **and** the rescuer fully opens the mouth and throat by tilting the head back and lifting the chin, the fluids or obstruction can pass back down into the lower air passages leading to the lungs and cause further obstruction to the lungs.

If there is a visible obstruction, the correct procedure is to roll the casualty into the recovery position (on their side) and then, with their head facing downwards, gently extend their head and neck to open the mouth and airway to allow any secretions to drain downwards out of the mouth. The rescuer may need to assist by sweeping the inside of the mouth with clothing, tissues or anything soft that is readily available.

It is not helpful to use an unconscious person's own fingers to clear their airway because this requires the rescuer to manipulate the victim's flaccid (floppy) fingers and multiple relaxed joints, which have no muscle tone or control, to try to reach into the back of the victim's own mouth and clear debris. The idea seems far more manageable than the practical reality of fumbling with floppy fingers inside the confined space of a mouth, plus it takes too much precious time.

The focus should be on clearing the airway quickly. Minimal time should be spent on rolling the casualty and draining the airway because any unnecessary delay during cardiac arrest can reduce the victim's chance of survival. When the airway is clear, the unconscious victim is then quickly rolled onto their back and, at that point, the rescuer needs to place one hand on the victim's forehead and the other hand on the chin and simultaneously push the head backwards while lifting the chin up. This action will lift the tongue away from the back of the throat and open up the airway to the lungs.

Infants and children

The same procedure is followed for a child – the head and chin are lifted in a similar fashion to a sniffing position. For an infant under 12 months, the head is *not* tilted. An infant's airways and membranes are small, soft and underdeveloped and their neck muscles are weak with poor muscle tone. Tilting the head and flexing the neck can actually cause a blockage by closing the soft air passages instead of opening them. So with an infant, it is imperative to gently clear the airway and then lay the infant flat with their head in a neutral position. This means that the infant's head is flat on the surface and not flexed or extended. Gently support the chin and do not move the head backwards.

Swallowing the tongue – an old wives' tale

The tongue is a muscle which is anchored at the floor of the mouth in front of the throat passages. When someone is unconscious, they lose muscle tone and are completely relaxed. If they are lying flat, the relaxed tongue flops against the back of the throat and blocks the airway. This reaction has been enshrined in folklore as having 'swallowed' the tongue.

The reality is that the tongue stays where it has always been and cannot be swallowed – it is just pushed against the soft structures at the back of the throat and this obstructs the airway. Tilting the casualty's head back and lifting the chin up opens the airway and lifts the tongue from the back of the throat.

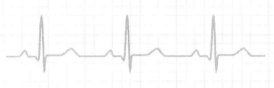

CHAPTER 25

CHECK FOR BREATHING

*'Breath is the finest gift of nature. Be grateful to the
supreme for this wonderful gift.'*

AMIT RAY

The next step in the DRSABCD emergency action plan (EAP) is to keep
the airway open and check whether the casualty is breathing by using
the 'look, listen and feel' technique. The rescuer can quickly determine if
the casualty is not breathing or is not breathing normally: at first glance,
they do not look well, they are pale and usually the skin changes colour
rapidly, turning dusky, blue or purple (*cyanosis* – pronounced 'sigh-uh-
noh-sis'). These are tell-tale signs that the casualty is in serious trouble.

Breathing may have stopped altogether or there may be abnormal
breathing – shallow, irregular, gasping (agonal) or noisy gurgling
breaths. In the first moments after a cardiac arrest, the casualty may
be taking infrequent, slow and noisy gasps as well as making sounds of
gurgling or sighing. This type of breathing is ineffective as it does not
move air into or out of the lungs, so the casualty should be treated as if
they are not breathing. Gasping breathing should never be regarded as
normal. It is also not uncommon for someone in cardiac arrest to appear
to be fitting or in spasm. Anything that appears abnormal probably is
and cardiopulmonary resuscitation (CPR) is most likely required after
phoning emergency medical services (EMS).

Rescuers do not look for pulses in an unconscious person

It is no longer recommended that rescuers search for a pulse when
someone collapses because if the person is in cardiac arrest, they do not

have a normal heartbeat; therefore, they will not have a pulse or blood pressure to circulate blood and oxygen. Most people are not skilled in looking for a pulse and critical time is wasted when inexperienced rescuers try to find a pulse, not realising there is nothing to find. In the past, too much time was lost before starting emergency rescue procedures. The easier, faster and more reliable method is to check whether the casualty is breathing.

The reality is that breathing and heartbeats (pulse) go hand in hand. In other words:

- Someone who does not have a pulse does not have a normal heartbeat and so cannot be breathing.
- Someone who is not breathing either does not have a pulse or will not have a pulse for much longer, if they do not start breathing again.

The latter occurs in situations such as drug overdose, suffocation, choking, drowning or any situation when the airway has been obstructed and breathing stops. The heart may still be beating at first but will quickly stop if breathing does not resume.

Resuscitation guidelines were changed in 2006 to reduce time lost and to speed up the rescue of someone who has stopped breathing. Any delay in starting CPR and providing defibrillation dramatically reduces the likelihood of survival. So the uncertainty associated with looking for a pulse was replaced with checking whether the victim was breathing which is easier and more reliable to assess.

Look, listen and feel

To check breathing the rescuer is quickly:

1. **Looking** for signs of breathing. Is the chest moving? Are the lips or cheeks moving with each breath? Are the lips turning blue? Does the victim's skin look a normal colour?
2. **Listening** for breathing. Facing towards the victim's chest, the rescuer puts their ear close to the victim's mouth and nose to listen for any air movement in or out of the mouth.

3.   **Feeling** for movement of air against the rescuer's cheek while they listen, also feeling for chest movement by placing one hand gently on the victim's chest.

This process should take no more than 10 seconds. It is important to remember that young children can breathe with shallow irregular breaths and with more tummy movement than chest movement.

If the casualty is breathing

If the casualty is breathing normally but is unconscious, roll them onto their side into the recovery position to protect and maintain an open airway. Continue to monitor them by observing that they are still breathing normally. Perform a secondary survey to check for any injuries or bleeding and make sure help is on the way.

Emergency call centre operators can assist in this assessment of breathing by asking the rescuer to put their hand on the patient's belly and let the operator know each time it rises. If there is more than seven seconds between rises (which is less than nine breaths per minute), the patient's breathing is ineffective and the operator will advise the rescuer in beginning CPR immediately.

If the casualty is not breathing

Anyone, child or adult, who is unconscious, not responsive, turning blue and is either not breathing or not breathing normally needs CPR urgently, commencing with 30 compressions, and defibrillation if an AED is available.

It is critical to start CPR immediately. Only leave the casualty to call for help when there is no other option available. If there is more than one rescuer, start CPR and ask someone else to send for help and get the AED.

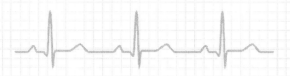

COMPRESSIONS

'There are no random acts ... We are all connected ...
You can no more separate one life from another than you
can separate a breeze from the wind ...'

MITCH ALBOM

When a casualty is unconscious, unresponsive and is not breathing or not breathing normally, they are in cardiac arrest and, after the rescuer sends for help, cardiopulmonary resuscitation (CPR) must commence without delay.

The purpose of chest compressions is to simulate the pumping or squeezing action of the heart to maintain circulation of blood and oxygen to the vital organs until a normal heart rhythm can be restored with defibrillation. Pushing down and compressing the chest squeezes the heart between the breastbone and the spine or backbone. This squeezing action forces blood out of the heart into the circulation and maintains the flow of oxygenated blood to the heart muscle, brain and other vital organs.

CPR buys the victim time until a defibrillator can be applied.

The evidence gathered internationally on survival rates from cardiac arrest supports the critical components of high-quality CPR to be:

- rate of 100–120 compressions per minute
- minimal interruptions in chest compressions
- depth of compressions depends on size of chest
  - » adult 4–5 cm or one-third depth of chest
  - » child one-third depth of chest

- allow full chest recoil without leaning on chest between compressions
- avoid excessive blowing of air (ventilation) – no more than 10–12 breaths per minute.[107]

Position of hands during compressions

The breastbone (sternum) lies in the centre of the chest and connects the ribs to the vertebral column (spine or backbone) on either side to form the rib cage. The heart lies behind the breastbone between the lungs, protected within the bony structure of the rib cage. The position of the hands during compressions is vitally important because, when the rescuer presses down, it is critical that the pressing movement pushes the breastbone down onto the heart and squeezes the muscle chambers which contain the blood. The squeezing action forces the blood volume contained in the heart to be pushed out under pressure to the lungs and into the circulation.

When the rescuer releases the pressure on the chest after each compression, the chest wall and rib cage rebound or expand. This helps the circulating blood return to the heart and lungs, ready for the next push of blood volume. This recoil movement also creates alternating positive and negative pressures within the chest cavity; in other words, pushing down on the chest creates pressure (positive) inside the chest cavity and releasing the compression eases the pressure (negative). The changes in pressure create a type of suction which passively draws some air from the atmosphere into the lungs, similar to the action of bellows. In addition, the changing pressures within the chest cavity assist the flow of blood into and out of the heart and lungs.

Leaning on the chest between compressions must be kept to a minimum. Human studies have shown that a majority of rescuers performing CPR often lean (put pressure) on the victim's chest between compressions but this does not allow the chest to recoil and expand fully. Leaning on the chest is known to reduce the blood flow in the heart and can also decrease the return of blood to the heart. If there is less blood being returned to the heart, the volume of blood that is expelled into the circulation with each compression will also reduce.[108]

Pushing down with the heels of the hands in the correct position – on the lower half of the breastbone in the centre of the chest approximately level with the nipples – is essential for effective compressions. It is important to not apply any pressure directly over the casualty's ribs, upper abdomen (belly) or the bottom end of the bony sternum (breastbone) because placing the hands incorrectly has the potential to fracture ribs or cause damage to internal abdominal organs. The ribs at the lower end of the rib cage are 'floating', meaning they are not connected to the end of the breastbone. It is possible to cause injury if compressions are performed too low and these lower ribs break and puncture abdominal organs. Compressions are also inefficient when the hands are placed too low because the heart is not being squeezed effectively.

If a rib fracture is heard (a cracking sound), simply reposition the hands over the sternum and keep going. A broken rib will heal if the victim can be recovered from the cardiac arrest.

It is also important to maintain straight arms with locked elbows, using the action of the hips and shoulders (not the back) to concentrate the power of the compressions through the heels of the hands. If the hands and fingers are spread out across the chest, the force of the compressions will also be spread across the chest and the compressions directly over the heart will be less forceful and less effective.

Significant power and energy are required to perform effective compressions, and performing CPR can be exhausting. Correct technique enables the rescuer to continue for longer and achieve more effective circulation of blood, increasing the likelihood of survival.

Why the number and rate of compressions have changed

Changes made to resuscitation guidelines, with respect to the number and speed of compressions delivered per minute, are based on evidence gathered internationally. When any changes are introduced, the focus is on improving survival outcomes. These changes do not mean that protocols that were recommended in the past were wrong; it just means that contemporary evidence supports updating the protocols to achieve better outcomes and a higher rate of successful recovery.

The international evidence on increased likelihood of survival currently supports that cycles of 30 compressions followed by 2 rescue breaths is the best sequence.

Previous practice was to start with rescue breaths and then follow with 15 compressions. But as more and more statistical data was collected from around the world, evidence showed that maintaining circulation with minimal interruption of effective chest compressions during a cardiac arrest had a significant impact on improving survival outcomes. Much more emphasis has now been placed on minimising interruption of compressions with rapid, smooth changeovers between rescuers.

The sequence was updated and 30 compressions are now done between the rescue breaths. This results in less frequent interruptions and more effective circulation of blood.

Another rationale that prompted the change was that, until the moment of collapse, the victim was breathing normally. Therefore the victim initially has adequate levels of inspired (breathed in) air and oxygen in their system to sustain them for four to six minutes before their heart and brain cells would begin to be impaired.

It is now believed to be more critical, early in a cardiac arrest, to circulate oxygenated blood throughout the body with high-quality chest compressions than it is to breathe more air into the victim, when they don't need it immediately. So, to improve the victim's chances of survival and recovery, the emphasis was changed in 2006 to compressions first, alternating with 2 rescue breaths after every 30 compressions.

When to give rescue breaths first

The exception to this sequence is when a cardiac arrest has resulted from airway (respiratory) obstruction, such as drowning, smoke, fumes, choking or drug overdose. In these situations, the casualty has already suffered oxygen deprivation before the heart stopped and so may not have sufficient oxygen in the circulating blood. Therefore, initial rescue breaths combined with chest compressions are recommended. Sometimes, if the victim has not yet gone into full cardiac arrest, these rescue breaths can be sufficient to stimulate spontaneous breathing again.[109]

It is important to note here that a rescuer must always consider their own safety first and exercise caution, if there is a risk that they could inhale toxic fumes from the victim's airways when delivering rescue breaths.

Public response to the changes

When the Australian Resuscitation Council (ARC) altered the ratio of compressions to rescue breaths to 30:2 in 2006, there was a significant amount of public scaremongering including a newspaper article published in Sydney on 13 August 2006 with the headline 'Kiss of death – paramedics and lifesavers fear new resuscitation technique could kill patients'. The ARC, which is Australia's peak body responsible for developing resuscitation guidelines, was concerned that the article made a number of statements that were 'inaccurate, misleading and could be potentially harmful'. The ARC was prompted to issue a press release in response because the claims could 'cause unnecessary confusion and anxiety amongst the community'.

Some of these key issues have been discussed in Chapter 16 'Myth 4 – An AED could cause further harm or injury to the victim' but are repeated here for context and continuity. The following statements, in particular, were refuted by the ARC:

Claim – 'The speed of compressions will almost double'

Fact – The ratio of compressions changed from '15 compressions followed by 2 breaths' to '30 compressions followed by 2 breaths' which in fact resulted in an increase in the *number* of compressions delivered, with fewer ventilations in the cycle. The actual rate of compressions, however, remained the same at approximately 100 per minute.

Claim – 'Professional lifeguards and Paramedics fear the guidelines, which include not checking the pulse, will put lives at risk.'

Fact – As noted in Chapter 16 'Myth 4', the chance of correctly finding a pulse in a victim of cardiac arrest is 50:50, which is about 'as useful as tossing a coin'. If a rescuer misinterprets that a pulse is present and the victim who needs CPR doesn't get it, then the likelihood of survival dramatically drops. The risk for these victims is extreme. If they are unconscious and not breathing, CPR should be commenced immediately.

Claim – 'Carrying out chest compressions on someone who is alive with a pulse could interfere with their heart rhythm, provoke a cardiac arrest and ultimately kill them.'

Fact – The ARC stated that it was not advocating that chest compressions should be performed on all persons who collapse. However, it also confirmed that no evidence exists that chest compressions on someone who has a pulse will do them any harm or cause any heart rhythm disruption.

Claim – 'It could be disastrous if well-meaning first aid officers started compressing everyone who fainted on hot days or passed out from alcohol or drug use.'

Fact – The recommendations of the ARC are clear in that only victims 'who are unconscious, not moving and not breathing normally should receive chest compressions. Where the patient has merely fainted, they will still be breathing, so clearly chest compressions are not needed'.

The press release concluded with 'The ARC is somewhat surprised by the notion that some in the community believe that the ARC ... and every resuscitation council around the world, would recommend a practice that was harmful'.

(The full press release statement can be found in Appendix D.)

Rate and rhythm of compressions

Compressions need to be hard, deep and fast with a steady rhythm and at a rate of at least 100 (up to 120) compressions per minute. There is no benefit from providing compressions at a rate that is too fast because it fatigues the rescuer, decreases the depth of compressions and does not allow enough time for the heart to refill with an adequate volume of blood in time for the next compression. Compressions then become less effective, which leads to reduced perfusion (circulation) of blood.

At the March 2013 ARC meeting, a minor amendment was made to the Basic Life Support Training Guidelines as follows:

At a minimum, mouth to mouth rescue breathing must be taught and assessed in any training program. It is the position of the ARC that all participants undertaking Basic Life Support training should be taught and assessed in mouth-to-mouth as a minimum standard for rescue breathing.

According to the ARC guidelines, the gold standard of resuscitation is to provide compressions and rescue breathing in a ratio of 30 compressions to 2 breaths which is the equivalent of a rate of 100 compressions per minute if no rescue breaths are given.

In other words:

- If no rescue breaths are given, the rate of compressions is continuous at 100 per minute.
- If rescue breaths are given, then the rate of compressions is still 100 per minute but they are interrupted by 2 rescue breaths every 30 compressions. The rate remains the same, with rescue breaths replacing some of the compressions.

Five sequences of 30 compressions and 2 rescue breaths equates to two-minute intervals.

There should be minimal interruptions between compressions because keeping the heart squeezing and the vital organs supplied with blood is critical to the casualty's chances of recovery. So even when giving rescue breaths, these should be quick, no longer than one second each, with a rapid return to effective chest compressions.

If rescue breaths appear to be unsuccessful – they do not make the chest rise with each attempt – do not waste time working out why. Return immediately to delivering 30 compressions. Before the next attempt at rescue breaths, quickly check that the casualty's mouth is clear, remove any visible obstructions and ensure that there is adequate head tilt and chin lift to open the airway.

To minimise the interruption to compressions, do not attempt more than two rescue breaths each time before returning to chest compressions.

Depth of compressions

Compressions should be one-third of the depth of the victim's chest. What this means is: if we were to measure the depth of our chest from the front at the breastbone between the breasts through to the back between the shoulder blades, the compression depth is approximately one-third of that distance. Because we are all built differently and weigh varying amounts, this depth will vary from person to person but the rule is still consistent.

The reason for compressing one-third the depth of the chest is because the breastbone sits directly over the heart and it must be pushed down far enough to squeeze the heart muscle, forcing blood out of the heart, into the arteries and therefore into the circulation. If the compressions are not strong and deep enough, the heart does not get sufficiently compressed and so blood is not forced out of the heart in an adequate volume to maintain blood flow and oxygen supply to the vital organs such as the brain and heart.

Why remove that bra?

When performing CPR on a woman, it is possible to compress the chest wall with a bra in place, but it is not ideal. A bra holds the breasts forward so that when the rescuer performs compressions they are pushing through breast tissue first before getting to the breast bone in the chest wall underneath. Providing CPR is exhausting and rescuers need to conserve as much energy as possible; therefore, pushing unnecessarily against the breast tissue requires more energy and tires the rescuer more quickly. Pushing down on soft breast before getting to the breast bone also gives the rescuer a false sense of depth and compromises the quality of the compressions. Underwiring in bras can also present an obstruction and restrict the quality and depth of compressions. Effective CPR can only really be done on a bare chest so bras and undergarments that impede access to the chest should be removed.

Delivering compressions

This book is not intended to be a 'how to perform CPR' manual. All first aid training should be undertaken in an accredited course under the supervision of a qualified trainer. However, for reference purposes, it is useful to include a summary of the correct CPR technique:

- Kneel at the side of the casualty with knees comfortably spread either side of victim's shoulder.
- Place heels of both hands (with fingers interlaced) in the centre of the casualty's chest (use heel of one hand for a child or two fingers for an infant).
- Press straight down on the sternum at a rate of at least 100 times per minute (a little less than two compressions a second).
  The most recent recommendation at the Australian Resuscitation Council 2015 Spark of Life Conference is a rate of 100–120 per minute although this guideline has not officially changed.
- Perform 30 compressions to one-third depth of chest – PUSH HARD, DEEP and FAST.
- Interrupt compressions and give 2 rescue breaths of no more than one second each. If there is more than one rescuer, a second person gives the breaths to reduce interruption time.
- *Rescue breaths*
  » open the airway by tilting the adult/child casualty's head back and lifting chin upwards, allowing casualty's mouth to open slightly; flat or neutral head position for an infant
  » if an adult, pinch the casualty's nose closed; if small child or infant, cover their mouth and nose entirely with rescuer's mouth
  » ensure a good seal of casualty's mouth with rescuer's lips or use a face mask if available
  » mildly blow into the casualty's mouth for no more than one second
  » maintaining head tilt and chin lift, take your mouth away from the casualty and look for the rise and fall of the chest but do not waste time
  » give second breath using same technique, again no more than one second

- Return your hands or fingers quickly to the centre of the casualty's chest and then give the next round of compressions and breaths.
- Continue cycles of 30 compressions and 2 rescue breaths.
- Apply an automated external defibrillator (AED) as soon as it is available.
- Unless the victim starts breathing normally again, do not stop resuscitation to check for signs of life.

Effective chest compressions are directly linked to survival therefore it is imperative to minimise interruption to compressions.

Even when an AED is applied, maintain focus on and minimise interruptions in chest compression. Do not stop to check the victim after defibrillation or discontinue cardiopulmonary resuscitation (CPR) unless the victim starts to show signs of normal breathing or responding, such as coughing, opening his eyes, speaking, or moving purposefully *and* starts to breathe normally.[110]

To reduce fatigue, if there is more than one rescuer, when compressions are interrupted every two minutes for the delivery of rescue breaths, another person can take over performing the compressions. Make sure the transition is smooth and swift to minimise disruption to the delivery of compressions.

Compressions only vs. compressions with rescue breaths

Guidelines for CPR and emergency cardiovascular care are constantly being developed and periodically updated; however, survival rates for victims of out-of-hospital cardiac arrest (OHCA) are not optimal and have not improved significantly over decades.

There are some evidence-based views in the international resuscitation community that chest compression–only resuscitation results in a better survival outcome than chest compressions combined with mouth-to-mouth ventilation in those victims of OHCA who had a shockable rhythm when emergency medical services (EMS) arrived.[111]

Danger of rescue breaths that are too strong

Rescue breathing is not similar to the force needed to blow up a balloon. Excessive ventilation must be avoided.

Blowing excessive air too fast into someone who is not breathing can do more harm than good because it does not allow air to be released or expired before the next forceful rescue breath is delivered. This creates abnormal pressure in the chest and restricts blood vessels at a time when the blood vessels need to be open and effectively circulating blood.

Hyper-inflating or blowing too hard into a person's airway can also damage the lining of the lungs and can force air into the stomach. The muscles of someone who is unconscious are flaccid (relaxed) so it is highly likely that stomach contents will be regurgitated because there is no muscle tone to prevent it. If excess air is blown into the stomach, at some point the stomach will expand and eventually expel its contents. The risk is that the patient may then 'aspirate', which means acidic stomach contents may flow down into the lungs, which can obstruct the airway and seriously damage the lung membranes where oxygen is exchanged.

Why consider compressions-only resuscitation?

The recommendation to minimise interruption to compressions by providing compressions-only resuscitation came about because the traditional CPR approach for laypersons had two major drawbacks:

- Too many bystanders who witness an unexpected collapse are willing to call for EMS but are reluctant to initiate rescue efforts because they do not want to perform mouth-to-mouth assisted ventilation, particularly on someone they do not know, which means that the victim could die unnecessarily. However, bystanders are more willing to perform hands-only CPR which is dramatically better than doing nothing at all.
- There is evidence that interrupting compressions to provide rescue breaths during cardiac arrest has a detrimental impact on survival rates, especially when rescuers take too long delivering breaths and thereby slow the compression rate or blow too hard into the victim's airways.

Compressions only – 'pros'

Without CPR or any attempt at resuscitation, a victim of cardiac arrest has no chance of survival. Therefore, in order to improve bystander rescue participation and increase a victim's likelihood of survival, the resuscitation guidelines allow the recommendation of doing compressions-only or hands-only CPR, which at least artificially maintains blood circulation long enough for paramedics to take over. It was deemed better for the bystander to at least attempt compressions rather than do nothing at all. With compressions-only resuscitation there is no interruption to compressions, which can improve the chance of survival. Hands-only CPR achieves the best outcome when emergency services are able to arrive within the first five minutes after onset of cardiac arrest.

Compressions only – 'cons'

Although introducing compressions-only CPR has had a positive effect on the participation of bystander rescuers and survival rates when EMS are able to arrive quickly and take over, there are negative consequences too. The longer a cardiac arrest progresses without rescue breaths, the more the existing levels of oxygen in the victim's body become depleted. After four to six minutes the victim's oxygen levels are significantly depleted and continue to deteriorate until the arrival of advanced life support, that is, medical personnel who can provide assisted ventilation. This oxygen depletion and the metabolic changes it causes to vital organs could lead to damage and/or death of cells in the brain and heart muscle. The victim now has a reduced chance of full recovery without neurological deficits (brain damage).

One of the less well publicised benefits of CPR is that compressions create positive and negative pressures in the chest cavity, which cause some passive movement of air in and out of the lungs. If a rescuer performs compressions only, they are not stopping to deliver rescue breaths, and therefore they are also not lifting the chin every two minutes to open the airway. As previously explained, when the chest is pushed down, pressure is exerted on the lungs, pushing air out of the lungs. In between each compression, the chest wall rebounds or expands creating a bellows-like effect, which draws air into the lungs. The end result is that, even without rescue breaths, there is some passive residual movement of air. The problem, however, is that an unconscious person cannot maintain their own airway. If the casualty is lying supine (on their back), unless the chin is regularly lifted to open the airway, the tongue creates an obstruction, which impedes or prevents passive airflow into and out of the lungs.

Current guidelines

Resuscitation guidelines are constantly under review and as more evidence on survival rates is gathered internationally there may be a paradigm shift where compressions-only resuscitation becomes the recommended practice in the first few minutes after a witnessed cardiac arrest, during the period when the victim still has sufficient oxygen in their circulation.

According to the British Heart Foundation, research has shown that lay rescuers are more likely to commence hands-only CPR. However, providing rescue breaths in addition to compressions should still be the gold standard. The preferred and recommended CPR guidelines by the Australian Resuscitation Council are also to provide compressions and rescue breaths at a rate of 30 compressions to 2 rescue breaths with a minimum time disruption between cycles so that compressions are interrupted as little as possible.

It is a normal human response to prefer not to put one's mouth onto the mouth of a stranger. Therefore, if a rescuer is unable or unwilling to give rescue breaths, the provision of compressions-only resuscitation at 100 compressions per minute gives the victim a chance of survival. This is a better option than no resuscitation at all which gives the victim no hope.

Tunes with the correct tempo for CPR rate and rhythm

Despite the morbid, 'black humour' song titles, the following tunes and nursery rhyme are the right tempo, are readily recognised and easily remembered to help rescuers keep pace with the correct compression rate for CPR, if a metronome from an AED is not available:

- *Another One Bites the Dust* by Queen
- *Staying Alive* by the Bee Gees
- *Baa Baa Black Sheep* – two verses.

In 2012, to encourage more people to perform chest compressions, the British Heart Foundation even produced a satirical video clip, featuring Vinnie Jones demonstrating hands-only CPR to the tune of *Staying Alive*.[112]

When to stop compressions

CPR can be stopped in the following circumstances:

- there is imminent danger or it is unsafe to proceed
- casualty responds, starts breathing normally and colour returns; that is, signs of life return
- the casualty's airway becomes obstructed – quickly clear airway and continue CPR
- more qualified help arrives AND takes over CPR
- when AED instructs rescuers to 'stand clear' and during defibrillation
- the rescuer is physically exhausted and unable to continue
- casualty is declared deceased by a qualified/authorised person, for example, paramedic or doctor.

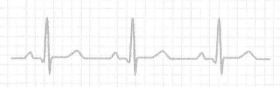

CHAPTER 27

DEFIBRILLATION

'The person who says it cannot be done
should not interrupt the person doing it.'

SOURCE UNKNOWN

The guidelines for cardiopulmonary resuscitation (CPR) have been in place for decades, but despite their international scope and periodic updates, there has been little improvement in survival rates in out-of-hospital cardiac arrest (OHCA) for victims of sudden cardiac arrest (SCA) who did not receive early defibrillation.[113] The development and availability of automated external defibrillators (AEDs) has significantly improved the potential for many lives to be saved.

While compressions are essential for survival, the most vital link in the chain of survival is early defibrillation. Its importance cannot be overstated. AED technology has dramatically progressed over the years and today's AEDs are safe, reliable, intelligent, effective, simple and easy to use. Despite the advances in technology, many impediments still persist so that AEDs are too often the missing link in the chain of survival:

- a lack of understanding of what a SCA is
- too many myths, fears and misconceptions inhibiting laypersons from using AEDs
- too few AEDs available in the community and workplace
- too few people are willing to use AEDs due to lack of knowledge and confidence
- insufficient understanding of the importance of uninterrupted compressions and rapid defibrillation

- a disparity between the law and AED technology (AEDs are not mandated inclusions in first aid kits)
- a lack of regulations governing the monitoring and maintenance of AEDs, as there are for fire equipment, to ensure that they are in working order.

The earlier a victim of SCA can receive a shock from an AED the greater their chance of survival. Hitting the heart muscle with a big dose of electrical energy is a bit like hitting Ctrl-Alt-Delete on your PC (or Alt-Command-Esc for the Mac users!). In nearly half of cases, a single early shock will cause the victim's heart to revert to a more normal rhythm with a palpable pulse and return of spontaneous circulation (ROSC), if defibrillation is given within a few minutes of the cardiac arrest.

The Australian evidence confirms that victims of SCA who are defibrillated by bystanders are three times more likely to survive than those who have only CPR because an AED is not available until emergency medical services (EMS) arrive.[114] Other overseas studies support this evidence.

In the 2014 *Consensus paper on out-of-hospital cardiac arrest*, the Resuscitation Council (UK), NHS and the British Heart Foundation (BHF) found that rates of bystander CPR and public access defibrillation (PAD) use in the United Kingdom are low because of:

- failure of bystanders to recognise cardiac arrest
- lack of knowledge of what to do
- fear of causing harm (such as breaking the victim's ribs) or being harmed (acquiring infection from a stranger when giving rescue breaths)
- fear of being sued
- lack of knowledge of the location of PADs
- no access to a PAD at the time of the cardiac arrest.

Reproduced with kind permission of the Resuscitation Council (UK)

Similar evidence of hesitancy, reluctance and lack of knowledge has been found in Japanese studies despite widespread availability of more than 350,000 AEDs in that country.[115]

As the chain of survival illustrates, a person is most likely to survive an OHCA if:

- the cardiac arrest is either witnessed by a bystander or the victim is discovered immediately after collapsing
- the bystander calls [local EMS emergency number] immediately
- the bystander delivers effective CPR without delay
- the cause of the cardiac arrest is due to a sudden 'shockable' rhythm disturbance caused by a heart attack or another heart condition, such as an inherited abnormality
- there is a public access defibrillator close by and bystanders use it without delay
- the EMS arrive very quickly (within minutes of being called).[116]

2014 Guide to automated external defibrillators

The Resuscitation Council (UK) and British Heart Foundation 2014 *Guide to automated external defibrillators* provides clear and succinct instructions on the application of an AED:

All that is required to use an AED is to recognise that someone who has collapsed may be in SCA and to attach the two adhesive pads (electrodes) that are used to connect the AED to the patient's bare chest. Through these pads the AED can both monitor the heart's electrical rhythm and deliver a shock when it is needed. The AED provides audible instructions and most models also provide visual prompts on a screen.

The AED will analyse the heart's electrical rhythm and if it detects a rhythm likely to respond to a shock, it will charge itself ready to deliver a shock. Some devices then deliver the shock automatically without needing any further action by the operator; others instruct the operator to press a button to deliver the shock (these are often referred to as 'semi-automatic' AEDs).

After this the AED will tell the rescuer to give the victim CPR. After a fixed period (two minutes in current guidelines), the AED will tell the rescuers not to touch the victim while it checks the heart rhythm and a further shock is given (if it is needed). Using an AED in this way allows the provision of effective treatment during the critical first few minutes after SCA, while the emergency services are on their way.

Modern AEDs are very reliable and will not allow a shock to be given unless it is needed. They are, therefore, extremely unlikely to do any harm to a person who has collapsed in suspected SCA. They are also safe and present minimal risk of a rescuer receiving a shock. AEDs require hardly any routine maintenance or servicing; most perform daily self-checks of (battery life, pad connection and system diagnostics) and display a warning if they need attention. Most AEDs currently offered for sale have a minimum life-expectancy of ten years. The batteries and pads have a long shelf-life, allowing the AED to be left unattended for long intervals.

These features of AEDs make them suitable for use by members of the public with little or no training, and for use in PAD schemes.

As well as having an AED on site (and people trained to use it) it is also vital that as many people as possible learn basic skills in cardiopulmonary resuscitation. This entails recognising that someone may have suffered SCA, calling the emergency services and then performing chest compressions and rescue breaths. This basic first aid will maintain an oxygen supply to the brain and other organs and make it more likely that the heart can be re-started by defibrillation. The priority in the early stages is to provide chest compressions, and if a rescuer is unable or unwilling to provide rescue breaths uninterrupted chest compressions should be given.[117]

(Excerpt from Resuscitation Council (UK) and British Heart Foundation 2014 Guide to Automated External Defibrillators): Reproduced with kind permission of the Resuscitation Council (UK)

Defibrillation protocols and procedures

Laypersons can be urban lifesavers and make the difference between life and death by defibrillating a victim of SCA long before professional help arrives. Rescuers should apply an AED as soon as possible and should not delay for any reason, unless there is danger. It is critical to the victim's survival that the rescue is smooth and without delay or interruptions. It is impossible to predict all the 'what if' scenarios, but having a procedural protocol in place is strongly recommended and highly beneficial.

An emergency plan that has been devised and prominently displayed helps rescuers to stay on task.

Multiple rescuers

A plan or checklist with tasks allocated to various people will increase the likelihood of a successful rescue. Tasks that could be assigned to rescuers include (not necessarily in order of priority):

- Ensure safety and clear area of potential dangers if safe to do so.
- Phone EMS for an ambulance and stay on the line with the operator.
- Control the scene, manage bystanders and direct activity.
- Start CPR immediately
  - » CPR needs at least one person, preferably two or more who can interchange the role of performing compressions to reduce fatigue
  - » changeover must be with minimal delay usually during rescue breaths every two minutes
- Protect casualty's privacy with screens if available.
- Prepare the casualty for defibrillation by exposing their bare chest.
- Retrieve the AED, take it to the casualty and apply the pads.
- Protect the AED from interference and damage
- Wait outside for paramedics to arrive and guide them to the rescue scene without delay.
- Contact family or next of kin if known.
- Keep track of time elapsed and prepare report of the event.

Single rescuer

The optimal rescue procedure is immediate and continuous compressions while the AED is being retrieved and set up. Starting compressions immediately keeps blood flowing through the heart, which means that defibrillation is more likely to be successful. However, when someone has a SCA, the best chance of survival is early defibrillation, so a lone rescuer is left with little choice about what to do.

AED easily accessible

Ideally CPR should be started immediately. However, if the rescuer is alone and an AED can be quickly accessed (within a minute or two), the rescuer should first call for help, then retrieve the AED and apply it to the casualty, before starting CPR.

AED not accessible

If retrieving the AED is going to delay compressions for too long, then the better option is to call for help, start CPR and hope that someone will arrive in time to get the AED. A Triple Zero (000) operator will always provide support and advice, but although it may be difficult, the best common-sense decision must prevail in these circumstances. Leaving a casualty in cardiac arrest without CPR for a prolonged period in order to retrieve the AED is very risky and likely to have a poor outcome. The problem is 'how long is too long?' The answer to that question is not certain so it is best to err on the side of caution and start CPR first, if an AED cannot be retrieved within a couple of minutes.

The AED utility kit

Most AEDs come equipped with an AED utility kit, which will typically contain:

- a pair of disposable nitrile synthetic rubber (non-latex) gloves
- a pair of trauma shears for cutting through a casualty's clothing to expose the chest
- paper towel or gauze for wiping away moisture on chest skin where pads are to be applied and clearing secretions from the mouth
- a disposable razor for shaving casualties with very hairy chests – only shave the two areas where the pads will be applied
- a face shield or mask for providing a barrier between patient's and rescuer's mouths during rescue breathing.

Preparing the casualty

Taking too long to prepare the casualty for defibrillation can significantly affect their survival. If there are two or more rescuers, CPR is continuous while others are phoning for help and quickly getting the AED ready.

Removing clothing

Clothing including bras must be removed to expose the casualty's bare chest. Ideally, metal items such as jewellery or piercings should be removed to avoid interference and burns from the shock. But removing metal items should never be allowed to significantly delay defibrillation.

If metal piercings cannot be removed, the casualty may receive a minor burn but that will not cause any lasting harm. If rescuers waste time trying to remove metal piercings, then the outcome could be much worse, that is, the casualty might not survive.

The American TV show *Mythbusters* found evidence that using a defibrillator on a woman wearing an underwire bra can lead to arcing or fire but only in unusual and unlikely circumstances. Exposed metal is not likely anyway because underwiring is enclosed within fabric. A bra with under-wiring is more likely to hinder effective compressions than to hinder defibrillation. Nevertheless, defibrillator pads should only be applied to bare skin, so all undergarments must be removed from the chest.

Removing excess chest hair
Skin is not a good conductor of electricity so the pads are coated with an adhesive conductive gel which conforms to the contours of the skin and provides an effective way to deliver early defibrillation. The conductive gel reduces resistance of the electrical current moving between the electrode pads and through the victim's chest.

In males, excessive chest hair can prevent the sticky gel on the pads from adhering properly to the casualty's skin. If the pads are not in full contact with the skin, the delivery of the shock might be less effective. Chest hair can also create air spaces between the pads and the skin, which can result in minor burns, so excess hair should be removed. If a disposable razor is available, rescuers should quickly shave only the small areas where the pads will be placed (not the whole chest) before attempting to apply the electrodes. If a razor is not available, application of the electrode pads should not be delayed. The pads should just be firmly pressed against the skin to get the best adhesion possible.

Applying the electrode pads
When the patient's chest is bare and the AED is turned on or opened, it will instruct the user to connect the self-adhesive defibrillation electrode pads. The pads have diagrams on them to help the rescuer correctly place the electrodes.

Rescuers should make sure that the patient's chest is dry, then remove the pads from the packaging, peel back the liner and press each pad firmly to the casualty's bare skin, as shown in the diagrams on the pads. One pad will go on the upper right side of the chest, under the collar bone, and the other pad will go on the lower left side of the chest, in line with the armpit.

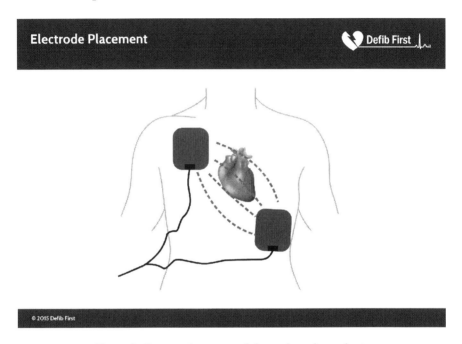

Electrode Placement

Defib First

© 2015 Defib First

Figure 8. Correct placement of electrode pads on chest

Placement of pads on chest
Rescuers should not place defibrillation electrodes/pads directly on the breasts of females. Always place the left-side pad on the casualty's chest wall under the breast to ensure that the shock travels directly through the chest to the heart and is not impeded by superfluous breast tissue.

Unless the rescuer is alone, rescuers should always continue with compressions while the pads are being placed on the chest. Once the pads are attached and the AED starts analysing the rhythm, everyone should avoid touching the patient so the AED doesn't pick up electrical interference.

It is not recommended or ideal to place the pads on the opposite sides of the chest (*upper* left and *lower* right). If this does happen, the AED would still detect the abnormal rhythms and defibrillate if needed; however, the quality of the shock could be compromised and less effective.

Whether or not a shock is advised

The pads must first be in place on the victim's chest and only then can the AED automatically analyse the electrical output from the heart and determine if a lethal shockable rhythm is present (either ventricular fibrillation (VF) or ventricular tachycardia (VT)). If the device determines that a shock is warranted, it will use the battery to charge its internal capacitor in preparation for delivering the shock. This system is not only safe (charging only when required) but also allows for a faster delivery of the electrical current.

When the capacitor is charged, a fully automated AED delivers the shock after advising everyone to stand clear. A semi-automated AED instructs the user to first ensure no-one is touching the casualty, and second, press a flashing button to deliver the shock.

When it is and isn't safe to touch the casualty

The AED will advise rescuers to stand clear when it is analysing the casualty's heart rhythm and delivering the shock.

As discussed in Chapter 15 'Myth 3 – An AED can shock someone who doesn't need to be shocked', rescuers should not touch the casualty when the AED is assessing the heart rhythm and delivering a shock. If the rescuer is touching the victim when the AED is analysing the heart rhythm, it can cause interference to the analysis. If the rescuer is touching the casualty when the shock is delivered, the shock shouldn't cause serious injury to the rescuer, but some of the electrical energy can be absorbed by the rescuer, dissipated and lost. This can result in a less effective shock for the casualty who actually needs it.

Resuming CPR after defibrillation

The longer that compressions are interrupted, the lower the chance that the casualty will survive, or survive without complications, such as brain damage. To give the casualty the best chance at recovery, compressions should be paused for no more than 10 seconds while a shock is being delivered. After the shock has been delivered, compressions should be resumed within five seconds.

Following the shock, the AED does not pause to re-analyse the casualty's heart rhythm to determine if the shock was successful. There is no evidence that re-analysing the rhythm gives any advantage and the delay in resuming compressions can compromise the casualty's survival. Not all victims start breathing spontaneously immediately after defibrillation so it is believed that the casualty benefits most if compressions are continued after the shock unless the victim resumes breathing.

As previously discussed, one of the 2010 International Liaison Committee on Resuscitation (ILCOR) – Consensus on Science and Treatment Recommendations was to minimise interruptions in chest compression when using an AED. The rescuer should not stop to check the victim after shock delivery or discontinue cardiopulmonary resuscitation (CPR) unless the casualty starts to show signs of regaining consciousness, such as coughing, opening their eyes, speaking, or moving purposefully *and* the casualty starts to breathe normally.[118]

After defibrillation, the AED will instruct the rescuer that it is now safe to touch the patient and to resume CPR, if required. The AED will wait another two minutes before analysing the heart rhythm again.

Tips for maintaining the right CPR rate and rhythm
Some devices use a metronome beat (regular pinging or beeping sound) to help the rescuer maintain the correct rate and rhythm for CPR. The metronome is set at the rate of 30 compressions then two rescue breaths. After 30 beeps for compressions the AED will instruct the rescuer to interrupt CPR, give 2 rescue breaths and then resume compressions.

The AED will repeat these instructions five times, that is five cycles of 30 compressions and 2 breaths, which is the equivalent of two minutes.

If the AED does not have a metronome, there are some well-known tunes that assist rescuers in maintaining the correct CPR rate and rhythm. As mentioned in Chapter 26 'Compressions', the nursery rhyme *Baa Baa Black Sheep* is the easiest to remember because reciting two verses is the equivalent of 30 compressions. (Note: there are those who are pedantically politically correct and have tried to change the colour in this rhyme to 'rainbow'. Doing so adds an extra syllable or 'beat', which changes the rhythm of the song. So, if you are uncomfortable using the word 'black', it doesn't matter which colour you use as long as it is a one-syllable word such as pink, brown, green, blue or red!)

The other previously mentioned tunes that have a CPR-friendly beat are *Staying Alive* by the Bee Gees and *Another One Bites the Dust* by Queen.

Some AEDs have added features such as sensors that assess the quality of the compressions and give real-time feedback on whether rescuers are providing good compressions or whether they should press harder or faster to improve the quality of the compressions.

Repeating the 2-minute cycle

The AED will re-analyse the victim's heart rhythm every two minutes to determine whether a shockable heart rhythm is still present. The AED will instruct either 'shock advised' or 'no shock advised'. If another shock is advised, the AED will repeat earlier instructions, automatically charge its internal capacitor and deliver the shock. (For semi-automated AEDs, the rescuer presses a flashing button to deliver the shock).

After the shock is delivered, or if another shock has not been advised, the AED will instruct the rescuer to continue CPR (if required) and the metronome (if included) will start again.

Throughout this cycle, the AED's only role is to detect and analyse a life-threatening abnormal heart rhythm and deliver a shock to correct and restore the normal rhythm. It does not, however, have eyes and ears and cannot determine if a victim is breathing or conscious. That is the rescuer's job.

Assessing breathing and conscious state if there is 'no shock advised'

If the AED instructs 'no shock advised' at any time after it analyses the heart rhythm, it will not tell the rescuers what rhythm it has or has not detected. However, the statement 'no shock advised' usually means one of the following:

- A normal heart rhythm has been detected and the victim is now breathing.
- A normal heart rhythm has been detected; however, the victim has still not resumed breathing.
- A 'shockable' heart rhythm has not been detected and the victim is still unconscious and not breathing.

It is the rescuer's job to be the eyes and ears to continually assess the victim's condition and determine the appropriate action, such as continuing CPR. If the victim commences normal breathing, CPR can be stopped because it would indicate that their heart has returned to a normal rhythm even if they are still unconscious. (Remember: it is not possible to breath, if the heart is not beating.)

If the patient is not breathing or not breathing normally, CPR is continued until the AED re-analyses the rhythm two minutes later and gives further instructions or until help arrives and takes over.

Performing a 'secondary survey' of injuries
Although the rescuer should perform what is known as a secondary survey, that is, check if the victim has any other injuries that require attention such as bleeding or broken bones, there is a first priority that always takes precedence over all other conditions – airway open and clear.

The primary survey is done to ensure that the airway is clear and assess if the victim is breathing. There is no point attending to secondary injuries (except, of course, severe haemorrhaging) if the airway is not open, because if the victim cannot breathe they cannot survive.

Post-defibrillation scenarios
While always keeping management of the airway and breathing in mind, there are only three scenarios that the rescuer needs to focus on after the AED has delivered a shock:

1. **Casualty is conscious and breathing.**
    The victim has regained consciousness in which case they must be breathing and have a pulse (heartbeat). After the drop in blood flow to the brain, they may be confused, disorientated

and sluggish, or possibly agitated and anxious. Therefore, it is important to:

a. calmly reassure them and explain what has happened
b. stay with them at all times
c. place them in a position that is most comfortable to them but not standing or walking
d. do not remove pads because AED will continue to monitor their heart rhythm at two-minute intervals and deliver more shocks if the patient relapses into cardiac arrest again.

2. **Casualty is still unconscious but has started breathing.**
   The victim is still not responding but there are signs that they have resumed normal breathing and their skin colour has improved. If the casualty is breathing, they must have a normal heart rhythm so the rescuer should:

   a. place an unconscious breathing person on their side in the recovery position
   b. ensure their airway is clear and open and mouth facing down
   c. stay with them to monitor airway and breathing in case they go back into cardiac arrest
   d. do not remove pads because AED will continue to monitor their heart rhythm at two-minute intervals and deliver more shocks if the patient relapses into cardiac arrest again.

2. **Casualty is still unconscious and not breathing or not breathing normally.**
   In this scenario, there are two possibilities. The shock has either:

   a. not reversed the abnormal rhythm
      or
   b. restored the normal heart rhythm but the victim has not yet resumed breathing (such as the case of Samantha at the Crossfit121 gym).

In both situations in Scenario 3, it is absolutely vital to:

- continue uninterrupted CPR and follow the AED prompts, for two-minute intervals
- not remove the pads because the AED will continue to monitor and record the heart rhythm and will deliver more shocks, if required.

Remember Samantha (Sam) from Chapter 19, who suffered a cardiac arrest at her gym?

In Sam's situation, after the AED delivered the first shock, CPR was correctly continued for two minutes. When the AED re-analysed her heart rhythm two minutes later, a second shock was not advised.

Sam was still unconscious and not breathing and CPR was continued until paramedics arrived shortly afterwards. With assisted ventilation from the paramedics, Sam started breathing spontaneously.

She had only required one shock to restore her heart to a normal rhythm but had remained unconscious and did not resume breathing immediately. This is a possible scenario that can occur after initial defibrillation and her rescuers performed a textbook perfect resuscitation. They just kept going with CPR until EMS help arrived. Had they not continued with CPR, Sam would have gone back into cardiac arrest because she was not yet breathing on her own.

Removing the pads

The AED will continue monitoring the heart rhythm at two-minute intervals until either the pads are removed or the device is closed. The pads are disposable and single-use only. While the pads are adhered to the casualty's chest, they are recording heart rhythms and other helpful data even if the patient has started breathing again. The data can later be downloaded and provides very useful information for medical management of the casualty after the event. Once the pads are removed, the AED can no longer detect and analyse a rhythm so it is imperative that bystanders do not remove the pads under any circumstances unless they are told to do so by paramedics (EMS) or more qualified medical personnel.

Downloadable event memory

Most AED units have an 'event memory' which stores the casualty's ECG (electrocardiogram of heart rhythms), along with the time the unit was activated and the number and strength of any shocks delivered.

Some units also have voice recording capabilities to monitor the actions taken by the rescuer which can be used later to ascertain if these actions had any impact on the casualty's survival. All this recorded data can be either downloaded to a computer or printed out as valuable feedback for medical management of the casualty. With this data, the manufacturer or distributing company is also able to evaluate the performance of the device and the effectiveness of both CPR and defibrillation. Some AED units even provide feedback on the quality of the compressions that were given during the rescue.

Implanted or internal pacemakers and defibrillators

It is recommended that rescuers avoid placing the AED's electrode pad/s directly over an implanted cardioverter-defibrillator (ICD) or a pacemaker (the battery pack is visible as a lump under the skin approximately 5–6 cm long). The medical default location (that is the usual site for placement in the chest) for ICDs and pacemakers is the left upper chest, so they are unlikely to be in the way of the AED pad, which is placed on the right upper chest. Sometimes, though, the implanted device has had to be inserted on the right side of the chest and it is best practice to avoid placing the AED electrode pad directly on top of it. Ideally, locate the pad about 8–10 cm away from the border of the implanted device.

Why do some people need a pacemaker?

I am so often asked if a pacemaker is the same as a defibrillator and whether defibrillation can damage a pacemaker. Someone with an implanted pacemaker has a problem with the heart's electrical system called bradycardia (*brady* = slow, *cardia* = heart; pronounced 'bray-dee-KAR-dee-uh') that causes the heart rhythm or pulse to be too slow to maintain normal blood pressure and circulation. The SA node that sets the pace of the heart beat is not doing its job properly and is too slow.

For some people, particularly fit, active, younger people, a slow pulse or heartbeat is normal and they experience no adverse symptoms. However, if symptoms are present and cause problems then the condition may need to be treated with an artificial implanted pacemaker. The most common symptoms that cause problems are:

- dizziness, weakness or light-headedness
- shortness of breath with difficulty exercising
- fatigue
- chest pains
- confusion, memory problems or difficulty concentrating due to reduced blood supply to the brain
- fainting (syncope) because the slower heart rate causes a drop in blood pressure
- heart failure and cardiac arrest (sometimes but uncommon).

What does a pacemaker do?
An implanted pacemaker takes over the electrical stimulation of the heartbeat when the natural pacemaker mechanism (SA node) becomes too slow. The battery pack for the artificial pacemaker is implanted under the skin below the collar bone and connects into the heart muscle via a wire or lead which detects when the heart rate drops below an acceptable level. The pacemaker then automatically generates a low-energy electrical impulse that causes the heart contractions to speed up to an appropriate rate that maintains blood pressure and adequate circulation and stops the symptoms. A pacemaker causes a slow heart rate to speed up but does not treat a cardiac arrest.

What's the difference between a pacemaker and an ICD?
Pacemakers and internal defibrillators or implanted cardioverter-defibrillators (ICDs) both have leads/wires inside the person's body which connect the device directly to the heart muscle so the heart can be stimulated if necessary, but pacemakers and ICDs are used for different purposes. A pacemaker increases a slow heart rhythm while an ICD stops a rapid and/or chaotic heart activity so the heart can restore a normal rhythm. A slow heart rate is not necessarily fatal; however, someone who needs defibrillation is in cardiac arrest which is fatal.

Is it safe to defibrillate someone who has a pacemaker or ICD?
If someone with an ICD suffers a cardiac arrest and requires external defibrillation, it is clear that their internal unit has failed. So the presence of an ICD should never prevent a rescuer from applying the AED on someone who is in cardiac arrest, that, is unconscious and not breathing.

The risk in placing an AED pad over an ICD or pacemaker is that electricity travels along the 'pathway of least resistance'. The electrical charge, therefore, would travel directly along the internal wire and concentrate the shock at the point where the wire inserts into the heart muscle. This has the potential to cause localised damage to the heart muscle.

The other risk is that the electrical energy could damage the internal pacemaker or ICD. If the implanted device is damaged and the casualty survives, it can always be replaced. There is no point replacing the implanted device if the casualty dies. Therefore, it is far better to defibrillate the casualty rather than to hesitate and not act. Best practice is to place the AED pads away from an implanted device, if possible.

Transdermal medication patches

If the victim of SCA has a transdermal (stuck on the skin) medication patch in place, the AED electrodes should not be positioned directly on top of the medication patch because this could cause minor burns or sparks and impede the delivery of the shock. If the patch is in the way of the AED pads, quickly remove it and wipe the area dry then apply the pads to the clean, bare skin.

Casualties in contact with water

For casualties lying in water (a pool, bath or the sea), it is necessary to remove them from the water before applying the electrodes. Electricity and water do not mix, so it is not safe to defibrillate someone who is immersed in water and it is impossible to perform CPR if the victim is not on a firm surface. On the other hand, there is no need to move the victim who is lying on snow or ice before applying the electrode.[119]

Risk only exists when the electrodes themselves are in contact with a body of water (rain not included). It could actually be an advantage if a victim was lying on snow or ice because medical research indicates that cooling a victim of cardiac arrest slows metabolism and cell activity thereby reducing damage to vital organs and enhances the chances of full neurological recovery.

Using an AED on children

AEDs may be used on children who are under 25 kg (55 lb) in weight or under eight years of age. If the AED is approved for paediatric use (that is, use on children), the adult pads must be disconnected and replaced with paediatric pads, which the AED is programmed to recognise. The shock delivered with paediatric pads is approximately 50% of the adult charge.

During AED presentations, the question is often asked about what to do if a child suffers a cardiac arrest and only adult pads are available with the AED or, alternatively, an adult has a cardiac arrest and only paediatric pads are available. (The former scenario is more likely to happen because an AED that is in rescue-ready mode will have adult pads connected by default. If adult pads are not connected when the AED is idle, it would display an error code and sound a regular beep alarm.)

In the unlikely event that these circumstances occur, the rescuer always needs to keep in mind that to do nothing in a cardiac arrest gives no hope of recovery. Therefore, although it is not ideal, if a child had a cardiac arrest and only adult pads were available, defibrillation would be done with the adult pads to at least give the child a chance of survival. The same premise exists for an adult when paediatric pads only are available – at least there is a chance of survival, if whatever is available is used. It must be remembered that paediatric pads are only used on children who are aged under eight years or who weigh less than 25 kg (55 lb) and this situation rarely occurs.

Another source of assistance and advice that is almost always available is the EMS operator or call-taker, who will offer guidance to a rescuer in any emergency situation.

Defibrillation by bystanders – in summary

Turn on the AED as soon as it is available and:

- Follow the voice/visual prompts of the AED immediately.
- Prepare patient for defibrillation
  » remove clothing
  » dry chest

» remove excess hair if necessary
- Attach the electrode pads to the casualty's bare chest as shown in diagram.
- Ensure nobody touches the casualty while the AED is analysing the rhythm and delivering the shock.
- Compressions must continue at all times except when AED is analysing the rhythm or delivering a shock.

If a shock is advised:

- Ensure nobody touches the casualty.
- Push the shock button as directed by the AED (fully automated AEDs will deliver shock automatically).
- Do not wait or check the patient after delivery of shock before recommencing compressions.
- Immediately resume CPR, using a ratio of 30 compressions to 2 rescue breaths, in time with the AED metronome (if present).
- Continue to follow the AED's voice/visual prompts which will automatically re-analyse the casualty's heart rhythm every two minutes.

If a shock is not advised and the victim is still not breathing:

- Immediately resume CPR, using a ratio of 30 compressions to 2 rescue breaths, in time with the AED metronome (if present).
- Continue to follow the voice/visual prompts of the AED which will automatically re-analyse the rhythm every two minutes.

Early advanced life support is a vital fourth stage of the chain of survival. Paramedics have advanced skills and drugs that can improve the victim's chance of survival, so the earlier they can arrive the better. However, bystander rescuers must never underestimate the most critical interval that has the greatest impact on survival is the time taken to apply an AED prior to the arrival of emergency medical services. Ordinary people can be urban lifesaver heroes.

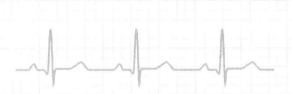

CONCLUSION

'I'd rather attempt to do something great and fail,
than to attempt nothing and succeed.'

ROBERT H. SCHULLER

And the beat goes on

Sudden cardiac arrest is a leading cause of death and there is no argument that early defibrillation within the first five minutes is the single most significant factor in the likelihood of the victim surviving *and* returning to normal life activities in the long term.

Minutes matter in a cardiac arrest and although on-the-spot defibrill-ation is the most vital link in the chain of survival, it is also the most frequently missing link. The problem is there are too few automated external defibrillators (AEDs) in the community and workplace and too few people willing and able to use them in those crucial first few minutes. Failure or hesitancy to act by bystanders when an AED is available contributes to poor survival rates and usually emanates from fear and a lack of knowledge and confidence.

Technology has advanced to the point that, these days, as well as CPR, defibrillation has become an integral part of an emergency first aid response routine, as it is the only proven way to resuscitate a person who has had a cardiac arrest. Competency in applying a defibrillator is now a regulated key element in first aid training. However, there are no regulations, guidelines or laws that require AEDs to be readily available in the same way that first aid kits, life vests and fire safety equipment must be in place, working and accessible.

No clinical skill is required to use an AED and all laypersons can respond to a cardiac arrest emergency effectively. As described in the Introduction, in July 2014 (winter and cold in Australia at the seaside) a group of strangers on a Victorian beach united as a team of urban lifesavers to combine their skills in CPR and locate an AED to save the life of Sean Purcell who had suffered a cardiac arrest.

Almost one year later, the survival story of another Victorian man, Jason Cripps, is eerily similar to Sean's, but this time in Perth, Western Australia. Both men were young, fit, athletic and out for a routine run. Unknowingly, both men were affected by viral illnesses which were later found to have contributed to their cardiac arrests. Both cardiac arrests occurred in out-of-the-way locations, which made their eventual recovery even more remarkable, due to the difficult access for paramedics and transport to hospital.

CASE STUDY: Jason Cripps

Jason Cripps is a 38-year-old husband and father of three children and a former Australian Rules footballer. He is currently the list manager for the Port Adelaide Football Club and was in Perth on Saturday 13 June 2015 to watch an Under-18 match as part of his recruiting duties. Jason set out with some colleagues on Saturday morning for a 5 km run. Only 200 m from the finish, he crouched down and collapsed in the dirt in sudden cardiac arrest.

Similar to Sean's rescue, another team of urban lifesavers, his colleagues and strangers, combined their efforts to give Jason another chance of life. One colleague, Michael Regan, and a doctor who happened to be walking nearby began CPR. Two ladies stopped and helped with the rescue. Other members of Jason's running group swung into action to help with CPR, send for help and guide the paramedics to the scene. The doctor was timing the incident and as 10 minutes of CPR passed, everyone was feeling anxious about Jason's likelihood of survival.

It was approximately 12 to 15 minutes before the first ambulance arrived. Two other ambulances followed and two defibrillation shocks were required before Jason started to show some signs of life. He was transported to hospital and maintained in a medically induced coma for three days. Jason's wife, Penny, flew in from Melbourne and was told of the real possibility that, if Jason survived, brain damage was likely and he might never be himself again. He had also developed pneumonia which complicated his already critical condition.

On Monday, three days after his cardiac arrest, Jason was brought out of the coma. He could follow instructions but had no memory of why or how he was in hospital. After six or seven days, Jason's recovery gained pace; his memory improved and he was walking laps of the cardiac ward. Specialists concluded from tests that Jason's cardiac arrest was caused by parvovirus infection and an implanted cardioverter defibrillator (ICD) was placed in his chest, just in case it happened again.

Jason's life changing near death experience has given him a greater appreciation of the importance of publicly accessible AEDs. He was lucky and blessed that a doctor and people who knew what to do were willing and able to be urban lifesavers. They kept his blood circulating with early CPR until the ambulance arrived with a defibrillator. Without the CPR, Jason would not have survived long enough to be defibrillated. However, it was the defibrillation that saved his life by restoring a normal heart rhythm.

No one can predict when they or another person will suffer a cardiac arrest and, in Jason's view, the widespread placement of easily accessible AEDs in the community will save lives when these unforeseen incidents occur. He believes it should be mandatory for AEDs to be located at all sporting events, businesses, shopping centres, restaurants and places where people gather.

Both Sean and Jason, along with Geoff Allen, Leigh Clarnette, Jenny Gifford, Samantha Jobe, John Ross and Michael Sukkar and the other case studies mentioned in this book owe their lives to the efforts of ordinary people who formed teams of urban lifesavers to maintain blood and oxygen circulation and provide lifesaving defibrillation. All have returned to their families and normal lives; their children still have their parents, however, their stories of survival, albeit inspirational, are the rare exception.

In the majority of cases, especially when there is a delay to defibrillation, such as Stephen Buckman who had also received good quality, effective CPR but could not be revived when a defibrillator finally got to him, the outcome is not usually a good one. It has been discussed earlier in the book that, in Australia, a sudden cardiac arrest is 590 times more likely to occur than a fatality caused by fire or smoke, 73 times more likely than drowning and 28 times more likely than a road fatality. Yet fire extinguishers are compulsory; life vests and buoyancy devices are mandated; seatbelt, mobile phone use, speeding and drink driving laws exist; but there are no laws mandating AEDs, despite defibrillators being the only means by which someone can be saved from a sudden cardiac arrest.

When you are diagnosed with cancer, you need a medical specialist to treat you and save your life. Survival rates of cancer victims are thankfully climbing with raised public awareness, increased research, earlier detection and improved medical treatments.

In comparison, when you have a sudden cardiac arrest, your life depends on the person standing next to you. Access to an AED and the reaction speed of bystander witnesses, before medical aid can reach the victim, determines life or death. It is imperative that the ordinary person knows what to do and feels confident and competent that they can save a life. All that is needed is the availability of public access defibrillators and education on how to use them. The more informed and aware ordinary people are, the more likely they will react quickly.

Although it is not necessary to have formal first aid training when applying an AED, it is best practice to be qualified in providing CPR and defibrillation. Lacking first aid training, however, should never prevent a rescuer from acting in a cardiac arrest.

Objectives of 'Back in a Heart Beat'

The objective of this book has been to bust the myths associated with sudden cardiac arrest and explain how ordinary people can safely use AEDs as well as to stimulate a shift in attitude in the community, workplace and government about the role of defibrillators in saving lives.

Defib First and not-for-profit Urban Lifesavers are committed to achieving this change through education and raised public and workplace awareness so that everyone knows how to recognise a sudden cardiac arrest and why they should apply an AED without delay.

The next objective of Defib First and Urban Lifesavers is to ensure that defibrillation does not remain the missing link in the chain of survival. Defibrillators are the key to restoring a normal heart rhythm. The more widely available AEDs are in the community, the earlier an AED is likely to be applied and the greater the chance of survival for the victim.

The goal is for every workplace, community organisation, club and public space to have a defibrillator as standard first aid equipment and ordinary people routinely trained to use them, without relying on designated first aid personnel to be available.

Businesses and government agencies could show leadership in this campaign with their commitment to corporate social responsibility and public safety. Placing AEDs in workplaces and community spaces, as well as providing training information sessions for everyone, would provide a priceless community service for a relatively low cost. The Asda retail chain has led the way in successfully implementing a public access defibrillation program at all of their UK stores and lives have been saved as a result.

Construction organisations could also take a responsive and responsible leading role by installing AEDs in another logical place – every elevator of a high-rise building. Municipal councils could locate AED emergency towers on street corners, in recreational reserves and on running and cycling tracks. Supermarkets, fast food outlets, convenience stores and petrol stations are ideal and easily identifiable locations. AEDs are commonplace in Japan and in some districts, they are available at over 90% of convenience stores.

Apart from the obvious benefit of saving a life, there are many other gains for the community and the workplace. Employee safety and security is reinforced as an important core value; more families are spared the grief and hardship from the loss of a family member; costs related to compensation, insurance and government welfare are saved; productivity losses are avoided; potential compliance, liability, and governance risks are minimised. The most important benefit, however, is peace of mind.

The ultimate goal is to bring about legislative change so that AEDs become mandatory equipment in first aid kits and regulations are put in place to ensure the AEDs are routinely serviced (as already applies to fire extinguishers) to maintain them in working order.

Defib First and Urban Lifesavers encourage everyone to learn first aid to build knowledge and confidence, or at the very least, attend an information session on how and why to apply an AED, which would minimise uncertainty and reduce delays.

Everyone can become an ambassador for change by starting the conversation and gathering your friends and family together for a training 'party' in your home or encouraging your employer or colleagues at work, club or association to get a group together to learn more.

Minutes matter in a sudden cardiac arrest and tens of thousands of victims do not need to die, if only we can get the message across that anyone can be an urban lifesaver – they just need to know how! There could be no greater reward than to save the life of another person.

> *I am only one,*
> *But still I am one.*
> *I cannot do everything,*
> *But still I can do something;*
> *And because I cannot do everything,*
> *I will not refuse to do the something that I can do*

EDWARD EVERETT HALE

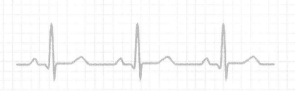

ABOUT THE AUTHOR

Anne Holland, owner and founder of Defib First and not-for-profit Urban Lifesavers, lives in bayside Melbourne, Australia. An experienced public speaker, presenter and trainer, Anne specialises in educating ordinary people to be Urban Lifesavers so that they have the confidence and knowledge to take the extraordinary action to restore the life of someone suffering a sudden cardiac arrest by applying an automated external defibrillator (AED) without fear or hesitation.

Anne is a Division 1 registered nurse with postgraduate coronary care qualifications and twenty years of experience in post-anaesthetic critical care. She is an accredited first aid trainer, a nurse immuniser and former lecturer at TAFE. She has worked as a triage nurse with the national Nurse-on-Call service, as an interventional medical imaging nurse, and as a program practitioner for a remedial intervention program treating cerebellar development delay.

She also works in government, private and corporate sectors providing medical assessment and immunisation services, data collection for clinical trials, and intravenous infusion delivery of lifesaving medication for patients in their homes and educating patients with chronic illnesses on how to self-inject their medications at home.

Anne's unique combination of specialised knowledge underpins her business, Defib First and her vision for not-for-profit Urban Lifesavers. She is a passionate advocate for education to raise workplace and community awareness of the use of AEDs, in order to remove fear and empower others to take immediate action to potentially save a life. Urban Lifesavers has been established to promote a national awareness campaign about the critical role that bystanders play in saving the life of someone suffering a cardiac arrest by applying an AED without waiting for paramedics to arrive.

Most importantly of all, however, Anne represents those who have experienced the grief and trauma caused by the loss of a beloved family member. Anne's husband, Paul, and father of their five children, did not survive a cardiac arrest in 2008. So she can speak with both personal and professional authority on the devastating grief and impact of cardiac arrest which touches two out of three families.

Anne's vision is to:

- bust the myths, fears and misconceptions related to sudden cardiac arrest and defibrillators
- educate the community on how to respond to sudden cardiac arrest
- promote increased numbers of AEDs in places where large numbers of people gather
- implement distribution of AEDs to workplaces and educate employees on how to apply them
- campaign for a minimum legislated standard requiring AEDs to be located within workplaces.

Minutes matter in a sudden cardiac arrest.
Anyone can be an Urban Lifesaver – they just need to know how.

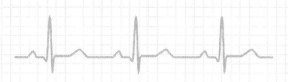

APPENDIX A – JOINT STATEMENT ON EARLY ACCESS TO DEFIBRILLATION

2012 Update to the 2002 statement:

A joint statement on
EARLY ACCESS TO DEFIBRILLATION

St John Ambulance Australia
Australian Resuscitation Council
National Heart Foundation of Australia

Key Recommendations

St John Ambulance Australia, the Australian Resuscitation Council and the National Heart Foundation of Australia call on the federal, state and territory governments to support early access to defibrillation through the following recommendations:

- Increase the number of automated external defibrillators (AEDs) that are accessible in places where large amounts of people frequent, such as train stations, casinos, sporting arenas, shopping centres, fitness centres, schools etc. and develop corresponding first responder programs that support their use.
- Develop appropriate performance monitoring and feedback mechanisms which evaluate the ongoing effectiveness of EAD first responder programs.
- Build community confidence in the use of AED through the implementation of community awareness campaigns that highlight both the misconceptions and benefits of prompt AED

use. This should be further supported by campaigns which alert people to the warning signs of heart attack and the importance of an early response by calling Triple Zero (000)

- Mandate the registration of all private and publically accessible AEDs, at the time of purchase, with local emergency service providers (i.e. the ambulance service) and Triple Zero (000) call centres.
- Develop a minimum standard to regulate the deployment of AEDs within large workplaces (over 200 employees) and to train employees in both AED use and CPR.

Introduction

It is estimated there are approximately 30,000 cases of sudden cardiac arrest within Australia each year[1], with the majority occurring out of hospital, and many as a result of an underlying acute coronary event. Raising awareness of heart attack warning signs and the importance of a prompt response among the community is vital in reducing time to definitive treatment for heart attack, with the Heart Foundation/Cardiac Society of Australia New Zealand – Guidelines for the management for Acute Coronary Syndromes (2006) recommending prompt activation of emergency medical services by calling Triple Zero (000).[2] For sudden cardiac arrest, the chance of survival decreases by 10% for every minute the victim is in ventricular fibrillation.[3] A sudden cardiac arrest is eminently treatable with prompt cardiopulmonary resuscitation (CPR) and early defibrillation.4 Early access to defibrillation (EAD) for sudden cardiac arrest is a vital link in the universally recognised 'chain of survival,' as the time taken to defibrillation is a key predictor of survival.

Within Australia, the concept of lay persons having access to and using automated external defibrillators (AEDs) for out-of-hospital sudden cardiac arrest has gained increasing support, as a result of its effectiveness in saving lives. However, more can be achieved by taking a systematic approach to the implementation of AED in the community providing greater access to and use of these devices for cardiac arrest.

ANNE HOLLAND – BACK IN A HEART BEAT

Systems of care for early access defibrillation

'System-based' approaches that reduce delay to medical treatment for time-critical emergencies, such as heart attack, have been implemented across various jurisdictions with excellent outcomes.[5][6] The success of these strategies has largely been dependent upon appropriate leadership and collaboration across health care services, clinical networks and government departments.[7] Similar, system-based approaches can be adopted to support early access to defibrillation and improve survival, including:

- Development and implementation of community-based first responder programs in high volume places
- Monitoring and evaluation of first responder programs
- Publically accessible AEDs registered with local emergency services

First responder programs

In Australia, as with other countries around the world, first responder programs aimed at reducing the time to defibrillation have been successfully implemented. Such programs involve the use of AEDs by fire fighters, police, security staff and volunteer first aiders from AED host organisations. These programs are linked with local emergency services to ensure the time to expert care is minimised. The first responder program implemented at the Melbourne Cricket Ground (MCG) is an excellent example of an effective systems approach to early defibrillation. This strategy has shown an 86% survival rate for cardiac arrest from first response to ambulance handover.[8] More recently, St John Ambulance Australia have coordinated Project Heart Start Australia (PHSA),[9] a comprehensive public access defibrillation strategy designed to raise awareness of early defibrillation among the community, train lay persons as first responders at AED host organisations and increase the breadth of AEDs within the public domain.

Outcomes from Project HeartStart Australia

To date, the program has approximately 400 publically accessible AEDs installed by St John Ambulance Australia across 120 organisations. Outcomes known to date from the PHSA program include:

- 40 reported activations of AEDs
- Of the activations where a shockable rhythm was administered and the patient transported to hospital, a total of 19 lives have been saved with many more anticipated over the life of the devices.
- The estimated cost-effectiveness of the PHSA project over a ten year cycle is $4343 per disability adjusted life year (DALY), which is considered very cost-effective based upon national benchmarks.[10]

The program has demonstrated that installation of AEDs, combined with appropriate training of lay persons can save lives and provide a sustainable benefit to the community.

Monitoring and evaluating first responder programs
Performance monitoring through appropriate data collection should be adopted to evaluate the ongoing use, capability and overall effectiveness of AEDs and associated EAD programs. Like all best-practice performance monitoring and feedback models, data collection should be integrated into existing systems and registries (where possible), culminating in national and state/territory-based performance monitoring and evaluation.

AED registration with emergency services
All AEDs purchased (independent of the purchase provider) should be registered with the appropriate local ambulance service by the exact street and site location. This information can then be loaded onto the Triple Zero (000) call centre's computer aided dispatch (CAD) system. When a Triple Zero (000) call is made by a bystander, the Triple Zero (000) call taker can immediately provide the caller with the precise location of the closest AED. This strategy can greatly reduce the time to defibrillation and is currently only occurring within Victoria.

'Busting' the myths associated with AED use
Making AEDs more accessible and increasing the number available will not automatically ensure that they are used. Training organisations in CPR and defibrillation play an important role in providing lay

persons with the confidence to use an AED in an emergency while importantly, busting the 'myths' of AED use. The perceived risk of doing 'more harm' and the fear of litigation are both common misconceptions among the general public and private sector, which unfortunately double as significant barriers to AED use and uptake, both in Australia and overseas.[11][12] AEDs are simple and easy to use and possess voice instructions for the lay rescuer to follow. Although training in the use of an AED is advisable for familiarity and confidence, a fully automated external defibrillator will not deliver a shock if it is not deemed necessary (unshockable rhythm detected), thereby making it easy for lay persons to operate in the event of a cardiac arrest. Furthermore, there have been no cases within Australia where a person or business has been sued for using an AED in an emergency situation. Most jurisdictions within Australia have 'Good Samaritan' legislation in place which protects lay rescuers from the risk of litigation when acting in good faith in an emergency.[13] *

* Specific legislation across Australian States and Territories referring to 'Good Samaritans' is in accordance with the relevant Civil Law, Civil Liability, or Wrongs Act for each jurisdiction.

Raising awareness among the community that it is safe to use an AED (both for the victim and the lay rescuer) is a key step to empowering bystanders to have the confidence to act as first responders, and ultimately reduce time to defibrillation. Early defibrillation (in conjunction with CPR), gives the best chance of survival, even if administered by a lay rescuer. We encourage federal and state/territory Governments to take a leadership role in raising awareness within the community on the importance, benefits and misconceptions of AED use.

Extending the breadth of AEDs in the public domain

Within Australia, AEDs are currently accessible in major airports and some major sporting arenas. AED locations should be extended to include other places where large amounts of people frequent, including train stations, casinos, shopping centres, and other sporting arenas. Furthermore, AED's should be accessible in places considered high risk of a sudden cardiac arrest such as health and fitness centres, sporting clubs,other registered clubs (i.e. senior citizens), major events and across settings with employees, students, or clients with known risk of heart attack. Some jurisdictions are acknowledging the importance of early access to defibrillation in settings considered 'high-risk,' with the Western Australian Government considering legislation that would make the installation of AEDs into commercial fitness centres mandatory.[14] Although regular physical activity clearly reduces risk of acquiring cardiovascular disease, evidence suggests heavy physical exertion in a small proportion of people may be a 'trigger' for an acute coronary event and subsequent cardiac arrest.[15]

Develop a minimum standard governing AED uptake within the workplace

To foster the uptake of AEDs within the workplace, a minimum standard should be developed which clearly outlines AEDs as a key component of workplace occupational health and safety. No minimum standard for AEDs within the workplace currently exists within Australia. A new national first aid code of practice for workplace health and safety is currently being drafted. The code of practice outlines first aid requirements across various workplace settings, including the implementation of AEDs in workplaces with large numbers of employees. However, this draft first aid code of practice is effectively a guideline only and falls short of setting mandatory minimum requirements. A minimum standard for AEDs governing larger workplaces (i.e. minimum 200 employees) could encompass the following areas (similar to that of fire extinguisher regulation):

- Accessibility (i.e. location and height)
- Visibility
- Maintenance
- Minimum number of staff trained in AED use

Regular training of workplace staff in CPR and AED use should become standard organisational best practice. We encourage workplaces within Australia to pro-actively consider and assess the efficacy of AED implementation within their own settings. Furthermore, workplaces are increasingly being identified as avenues for health promotion and health education for the workforce in Australia (the Victorian Work Health program is an example of this approach). As a result, the Heart

Foundation has developed a 'Warning signs of heart attack education program' which includes a suite of resources supporting workplaces to implement warning signs messages into new and existing workplace health programs.[16]

Conclusion

Early access to defibrillation is vital to improving outcomes from sudden cardiac arrest. AEDs in the public domain (such as major airports and some sporting stadiums) have been shown to reduce time to defibrillation and save lives. Furthermore, first responder programs are effective in reducing time to defibrillation and provide a smooth transition to pre-hospital emergency medical services.

St John Ambulance Australia, the Australian Resuscitation Council and the Heart Foundation call upon the federal and state and territory governments to take the lead in developing and implementing early access defibrillation policy, ensuring the 30,000 Australians who suffer out-of-hospital cardiac arrest every year are given the best chance of survival.

References

1   Estimate provided by the Australian Resuscitation Council.

2   JC Finn, JH Nick Bett, TR Shilton, et al. 2007 Patient delay in responding to symptoms of possible heart attack: can we reduce time to care? MJA 2007; 187 (5): 293–298

3   Sunde K, Jacobs I, Deakin CD, Hazinski MF, Kerber RE, Koster RW, Morrison LJ, Nolan JP, Sayre MR. Part 6: Defibrillation: 2010 International Consensus on Cardiopulmonary Resuscitation and Emergency Cardiovascular Care Science with Treatment Recommendations. Resuscitation 2010; 81: e71–e85.

4   Australian Resuscitation Council … guideline …

5   I Meredith, A Hutchison, Y Malaiapan, et al. Prehospital 12-Lead ECG to Triage ST-Elevation Myocardial Infarction and Emergency Department Activation of the Infarct Team Significantly Improves Door-to-Balloon Times. Circ Cardiovasc Inter 2009;2;528-534.

6   AB Wilson, D Mountain, JM Jeffers, et al. Door-to-balloon times are reduced in ST-elevation myocardial infarction by emergency physician activation of the cardiac catheterisation laboratory and immediate patient transfer. MJA 2010; 193: 207–212.

7   Brieger D, Kelly A, Aroney C, et al. Acute coronary syndromes: consensus recommendations for translating knowledge into action. Med J Aust 2009; 191: 334–338.

8   Wassertheil, Keane, Leditchke. Cardiac arrest outcomes at the Melbourne Cricket Ground and Shrine of Remembrance using a tiered response strategy. Resuscitation 2000; 44: 97–104.

9   Project Heart Start Australia, cited on: www.sja.com.au

10   Access Economics. The economic and social contribution of St John Ambulance Australia. March 2010

11   Schober P, van Dehn FB, Bierens JJLM, Loer SA, Schwarte LA. Public Access Defibrillation: Time to Access the Public. Ann Emerg Med 2011; 58 (3): 240-7

12   Campbell Research & Consulting (Prepared for the Department of health and Ageing). An Evaluation of the Public Access Defibrillation (PAD) Demonstration, Final Report. August 2008

13   Australian Resuscitation Council. Legal and Ethical Issues related to Resuscitation Guideline 10.5 (updated July 2011).
     Accessed at: http://www.resus.org.au/policy/guidelines/section_10/legal_ethical.htm

14   Government of Western Australia, Department of Health. Proposal to introduce Automated External Defibrillators in Gymnasiums: Consultation paper. 2010

15   Strike PC, Steptoe A. Behavioural and Emotional Triggers of Acute Coronary Syndromes: A Systematic Review and Critique. Psychosomatic Medicine. 2005; 67: 179-186.

16   Heart Foundation. Warning Signs of Heart Attack Education Program. 2011

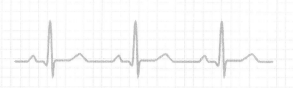

APPENDIX B – GOVERNANCE OF FIRST AID TRAINING IN AUSTRALIA

Australia's Vocational Education and Training sector

Vocational Education and Training (VET) enables students to gain qualifications for all types of employment and specific skills to help them in the workplace. VET is provided through a network of eight state and territory governments and the Australian Government, along with industry, public and private training providers. These organisations work together to provide nationally consistent training across Australia.

The providers of VET include Technical and Further Education (TAFE) institutes, adult and community education providers and agricultural colleges, as well as private providers, community organisations, industry skill centres, and commercial and enterprise training providers. In addition, some universities and schools provide VET.

The VET sector is crucial to the Australian economy, both for the development of the national workforce and as a major export industry.

Australian Skills Quality Authority

The Australian Skills Quality Authority (ASQA) (http://www.asqa.gov.au/) is the national regulator for the VET sector. ASQA seeks to make sure that the sector's quality is maintained through the effective regulation of providers and accredited courses.

ASQA regulates to ensure training meets the needs of industry by:

- ensuring risks to quality VET are well managed
- employing a strong compliance, auditing and monitoring regime and a range of escalating sanctions

- recognising the need for innovation and flexibility in VET.

In its regulatory approach, ASQA works to achieve a balance between the wider interests of Australian industry and Australian employers and the specific interests of the vocational education industry.

Australian businesses need a skilled workforce. Through the work of Industry Skills Councils in developing training packages, industry defines the skills required by the labour market. ASQA ensures that registered training organisations (RTOs) are meeting the requirements of these industry-developed training packages, so that VET graduates have the required skills and competencies for employment.

Australian Qualifications Framework

The Australian Qualifications Framework (AQF) (http://www.aqf.edu.au) establishes the quality of Australian qualifications and is the national policy for regulated qualifications in the Australian education and training system. The AQF was first introduced in 1995 to underpin the national system of qualifications in Australia encompassing higher education, VET and schools. AQF incorporates the quality assured qualifications from each education and training sector into a single, comprehensive national qualifications framework.

In Australia, education and training is a shared responsibility of all federal, state and territory governments. Education, training and employment ministers collectively own and are responsible for the AQF.

Training.gov.au

Training.gov.au (https://training.gov.au/) is a joint initiative of the Australian and state and territory governments and is the official national register of VET in Australia. Training.gov.au is managed by the Department of Industry and Science on behalf of state and territory governments.

Training.gov.au is the authoritative source of information on:
1. Nationally Recognised Training (NRT) which consists of:
   - Training Packages
   - Qualifications
   - Units of competency

- Accredited courses
- Skill sets

2. Registered Training Organisations (RTOs) who have the approved scope to deliver Nationally Recognised Training, as required by national and jurisdictional legislation within Australia.

Data on training.gov.au is maintained by:

Industry Skills Councils (ISCs) and **Auto Skills Australia** [which oversee]:

- Training Packages
- Qualifications
- Unit[s] of competency
- Skill sets

Vocational Education and Training Regulators [which oversee]:

- Registered Training Organisation (RTO) details and scope information
- Accredited courses

Revised performance evidence – 'Provide cardiopulmonary resuscitation'

First aid training is a series of regulated units of competency within the Health Training Package (HLT) which is governed by the Community Services and Health Industry Skills Council.

A revised unit of competency 'HLTAID001 – Provide cardiopulmonary resuscitation' was released on 1 July 2013 to incorporate mandatory assessment of competency in the application of an automated external defibrillator (AED). The changes came into force on 1 July 2014.

Previous unit of competency 'HLTCPR211A – Perform CPR'

Before 1 July 2013, an employer with 10 or more employees was required to provide first aid–trained personnel who were competent in providing CPR until paramedics arrived and took over. At that time, the regulations for the first aid unit of competency 'HLTCPR211A – Perform CPR' only required the training participant to 'have an understanding' of what an automated external defibrillator (AED) was and how it worked. There was no mandatory training and assessment in applying an AED during a cardiac arrest nor was there any requirement for AEDs to be available during the training for participants to see how they worked.

From 1 July 2013 'HLTAID001 –
Provide cardiopulmonary resuscitation'

On 1 July 2013, the previous first aid training regulations and requirements were superseded. The new unit of competency 'HLTAID001 – Provide cardiopulmonary resuscitation', which all first aid personnel must complete each year, requires participants to be assessed and deemed competent not only in the performance of effective CPR but also in the application and operation of an AED. For participants to be assessed as competent, the training provider must have AEDs available for practical demonstration and the candidates must actively participate in operating them.

The performance evidence of HLTAID001 Release 4 requires:

The candidate must show evidence of the ability to complete tasks outlined in elements and performance criteria of this unit, manage tasks and manage contingencies in the context of the job role.

There must be evidence that the candidate has completed the following in line with state/territory regulations, first aid codes of practice, Australian Resuscitation Council (ARC) guidelines and workplace procedures:

- Followed DRSABCD in line with ARC guidelines, including:
  - » performed at least 2 minutes of uninterrupted single rescuer cardiopulmonary resuscitation (CPR) (5 cycles of both compressions and ventilations) on an adult resuscitation manikin placed on the floor
  - » performed at least 2 minutes of uninterrupted single rescuer CPR (5 cycles both compressions and ventilation) on an infant resuscitation manikin placed on a firm surface
  - » responded appropriately in the event of regurgitation or vomiting managed the unconscious breathing casualty
  - » followed single rescuer rescue procedure, including the demonstration of a rotation of operators with minimal interruptions to compressions
  - » **followed the prompts of an automated external defibrillator (AED)** [emphasis added]

- Responded to at least one simulated first aid scenario contextualised to the candidate's workplace/community setting including:
  » demonstrated safe manual handling techniques
  » provided an accurate verbal or written report of the incident.

Assessment Requirements for HLTAID001 Provide cardiopulmonary resuscitation, Commonwealth of Australia, Licensed under the CC-BY-ND 3.0 Australia Licence. Downloaded from: www.training.gov.au.

APPENDIX C – GOOD SAMARITAN LEGISLATION IN AUSTRALIA

State/ Territory	Legislation	Protection	Exclusion From Protection
ACT	*Civil Law (Wrongs) Act 2002, S 5*	Honestly and without recklessness	Liability falls within ambit of a scheme of compulsory third party motor vehicle insurance Capacity to exercise appropriate care and skill was significantly impaired by a recreational drug
NSW	*Civil Liability Act 2002, S 57*	In good faith	If the Good Samaritan's intentional or negligent act or omission caused the injury or risk of injury. Ability to exercise reasonable care and skill was significantly impaired by being under the influence of alcohol or a drug voluntary consumed. Failed to exercise reasonable care and skill
NT	*Personal Injuries (Liabilities and Damages) Act 2003, S 8*	In good faith and without recklessness	Intoxicated while giving the assistance or advice

QLD	*Law Reform Act 1995*	In good faith and without gross negligence	Protection of medical practitioners and nurses and other prescribed persons
	Civil Liability Act 2003 (Good Samaritan) Amendment Bill 2007	Defeated 4 Sept 2007	Was intended to protect all persons who rendered first aid
SA	*Civil Liability Act 1936, S 74*	In good faith and without recklessness	Liability falls within ambit of a scheme of compulsory third party motor vehicle insurance. Capacity to exercise due care and skill was significantly impaired by alcohol or another recreational drug
Tas.	*Civil Liability Act 2002, S 35B*	In good faith and without recklessness even if the emergency or accident was caused by an act or omission of the Good Samaritan	Does not apply to any act or omission of a Good Samaritan that occurs before the assistance, advice or care is provided by the Good Samaritan
Vic.	*Wrongs Act 1958, S 31B*	In good faith even if emergency or accident was caused by an act or omission of the Good Samaritan	Does not apply to any act or omission of a Good Samaritan that occurs before the assistance, advice or care is provided by the Good Samaritan
WA	*Civil Liability Act 2002, 5AD*	In good faith and without recklessness	Ability to exercise reasonable care and skill was significantly impaired by being intoxicated by alcohol or a drug or other substance and intoxication was self-induced

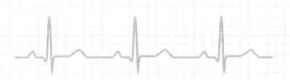

APPENDIX D – AUSTRALIAN RESUSCITATION COUNCIL PRESS RELEASE 2006

Press Release

"Kiss of Death – Paramedics and lifesavers fear new resuscitation technique could kill patients"

The Australian Resuscitation Council (ARC) has been made aware of an article that was published in the Sunday Telepgraph on August 13th 2006. The Council is concerned that the article makes a number of statements that are inaccurate, misleading and could be potentially harmful. It is unfortunate that these statements have been made as they cause unnecessary confusion and anxiety amongst the community.

The ARC is Australia's peak body responsible for developing resuscitation guidelines and comprises representation from various medical, nursing, ambulance and community organisations involved in the teaching and practice of resuscitation. The guidelines and subsequent recommendations are produced after carefully reviewing the scientific evidence, considering clinical experience and seeking input from the councils many member organisations. Updated guidelines were released in March 2006 following the most extensive international review of the resuscitation science ever undertaken. The ARC was part of this review process along with other resuscitation councils including the American Heart Association, the European Resuscitation Council and Resuscitation Council of Southern Africa.

Of particular concern to the ARC are the following statements that appeared in the newspaper article.

"The speed of compressions will almost double."
This is incorrect as the rate of compressions has always been 100 per minute. What does change is the number of compressions delivered, will increase as more compressions and fewer ventilations are delivered, when using a compression/ventilation ratio of 30:2.

"Professional lifeguards and Paramedics fear the guidelines, which includes not checking the pulse, will put lives at risk."
"Carrying out chest compressions on someone who is alive with a pulse could interfere with their heart rhythm, provoke a cardiac arrest and ultimately kill them."
There is no evidence whatsoever that performing chest compressions on someone who has a pulse will cause harm. In fact the recommendation has been for decades that chest compressions should be performed in unconscious children where their pulse is slower than normal. The same is often the case for unconscious adults who have slow pulse rates. This has been done without harm and docs not cause disturbances of heart rhythm.

"It could be disastrous if well meaning first aid officers started compressing everyone who fainted on hot days or passed out from alcohol or drug use."
The ARC is not advocating that everyone who collapses has chest compressions performed on them. What the council is recommending is that patients who are UNCONSCIOUS, NOT MOVING and NOT BREATHING NORMALLY should receive chest compressions. Where the patient has merely fainted they will still be breathing so clearly chest compressions are not needed. There is considerable evidence that when using the pulse check on someone who has suffered a cardiac arrest you have a 50:50 chance of correctly determining if a pulse rate is present or absent. In other words it is just as useful as tossing a coin. The greatest risk is to patients who need CPR but don't get it because the

rescuer believes the pulse to be present. In this situation the likelihood of survival falls dramatically.

It is interesting to note that while the guidelines were updated in 2006, the changes that raised concern in the newspaper article were part of changes made by the ARC back in 2000.

The updated guidelines have been endorsed by all members of the ARC. This includes St. John Ambulance, Surf Life Saving Australia, Royal Life Saving Australia, Ambulance Services throughout Australia, National Heart Foundation, Australian Red Cross, Cardiac Society of Australia and New Zealand, Colleges of Nursing and Colleges of Medicine including Emergency Medicine, Intensive Care, Surgeons, Anaesthesia and General Practice. The ARC is somewhat surprised by the notion that some in the community believe that the ARC, and every resuscitation council around the world, would recommend a practice that was harmful.

Further information can be obtained from the ARC website (www.resus. org.au) including the ARC guidelines and answers to frequently asked questions.

Associate Professor Ian Jacobs
Chariman

14th August 2006

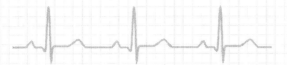

GLOSSARY

ABS – Australian Bureau of Statistics

ACLS – advanced cardiac life support

AED – automated external defibrillator

AF – atrial fibrillation – the heart's upper chambers 'quiver' but AF is not fatal

agonal breaths – gasping breaths (common in initial phase of cardiac arrest)

AHA – American Heart Association

alveoli – microscopic air pockets in the lungs where oxygen is exchanged

AMI – acute myocardial infarction or heart attack

ARC – Australian Resuscitation Council

arrhythmia – abnormal heart rhythm (pronounced 'ay-RITH-me-ah')

aspirate (lungs) – accidental suction of stomach contents into the lungs

asystole – cardiac standstill or flat-line heart rhythm (pronounced 'ay-sis-toe-lee')

atria – two upper smaller chambers inside heart that collect blood from lungs and the rest of the body and transfer it to the lower chambers (ventricles)

BHF – British Heart Foundation

biphasic waveform – two sequential shocks delivered to the heart via the AED's two electrodes/pad with each shock moving in an opposite vector/direction to the other

bradycardia – heart beats too slowly (brady = slow; cardia = heart)

cardiac arrhythmia – abnormal heart rhythm

cardiac refill – time interval between one heart or pulse beat and the next, when the heart refills with blood ready for the next contraction

cardiologist – doctor who specialises in heart conditions and diseases

casualty – someone who is injured or killed

chain of survival – series of early actions designed to improve the survival rate for people who have a sudden cardiac arrest – early access, early CPR, early defibrillation, early ACLS

commotio cordis – cardiac arrest resulting from a sudden blow or impact to the chest

CPR – cardiopulmonary resuscitation

CVA – cerebro-vascular accident or stroke

CVD – cardiovascular disease

cyanosis – purple or blue discolouration of the skin

defibrillator – device that delivers an electric shock to heart muscle to restore normal rhythm

EAD – early access to defibrillation

EAP – emergency action plan

ECG – electrocardiogram

electrophysiologist – doctor who specialises in diagnosis and treatment of heart rhythm disorders

EMS – emergency medical services

EPIRB – electronic position indicating radio beacon

fibrillation – chaotic quivering electrical activity of the muscle cells

GSM – Global System for Mobile Communications

HCM or HCOM – hypertrophic cardiomyopathy – disease of the heart muscle (cardiomyopathy) when the muscle is abnormally thickened (hypertrophy)

hemiplegia – one side of body is paralysed

hypothermia – lower than normal body temperature

hypoxia – body is deprived of an adequate oxygen supply

ICD – implantable cardioverter-defibrillator

ILCOR – International Liaison Committee on Resuscitation

layperson – a person not qualified in a specific profession

LQTS – long QT syndrome – an abnormal heart rhythm that can result in cardiac arrest

metronome – a device that produces a fixed regular beat or click

monophasic waveform – electrical waveform used in early defibrillators – shock travelled in one direction through the heart (from one electrode pad to the other)

MPDS – Medical Priority Dispatch System

myocardial – relating to heart muscle

NHF – National Heart Foundation

NHS – National Health Service in Britain

occult – hidden, with no symptoms

oesophagus – food pipe from back of throat down to stomach

OHCA – out-of-hospital cardiac arrest

OH&S – occupational health and safety

PAD – public access defibrillation

perfusion – circulation of blood

PPE – personal protective equipment

ROSC – return of spontaneous circulation, that is, detectable pulse

RTO – registered training organisation

SADS – sudden arrhythmic death syndrome

SA node – sino-atrial node – pacemaker node at top of heart that stimulates the heartbeat

SCA – sudden cardiac arrest

SCAF – Sudden Cardiac Arrest Foundation

SCD – sudden cardiac death

sinus rhythm – a normal heart rhythm or heartbeat which originates from SA node

sternum – breastbone in centre of chest

stroke – CVA – cerebrovascular accident (abnormality of blood vessel in brain)

syncope – fainting (pronounced 'sin-ko-pea')

tachycardia – heart beats too fast (tachy = fast; cardia = heart)

trachea – wind pipe through which air passes from the mouth/nose into the lungs

transdermal patch – adhesive patch of medication that is stuck to and absorbed through the skin

transthoracic impedance – resistance to electrical current through chest wall related to size of patient

TTY – text telephone/teleprinter/teletype/telephone typewriter – electronic device used by people with hearing or speech impairment that allows text communication over telephone landlines

VACAR – Victorian Ambulance Cardiac Arrest Registry

ventricles – two lower, larger chambers inside heart that receive blood from upper chambers (atria) and pump it to lungs and rest of body

VF – ventricular fibrillation – ventricles quivering or fibrillating

VT – ventricular tachycardia – ventricles beating too fast

WHS – workplace health and safety

NOTES

1   National Heart Foundation of Australia, '2014 Data and Statistics', [online – accessed 30 August 2015], <http://www.heartfoundation.org.au/information-for-professionals/data-and-statistics/Pages/default.aspx>.

2   ibid

3   National Heart Foundation of Australia, Media Release, 'Lack of direct action flags dire warnings for cardiovascular disease', 16 December 2014, [online], <http://www.heartfoundation.org.au/news-media/Media-Releases-2014/Pages/lack-direct-action-flags-dire-warnings-cardiovascular-disease.aspx> [accessed 10 January 2015].

4   Sudden Cardiac Arrest Foundation, 'Sudden Cardiac Arrest: A Healthcare Crisis' [online], <http://www.sca-aware.org/about-sca>, [accessed 30 August 2015].

5   National Heart Foundation of Australia, Media Release, 'Three in five women unaware of heart risk', 1 June 2013, <http://www.heartfoundation.org.au/news-media/Media-Releases-2013/Pages/women-unaware-heart-risk.aspx> [accessed 27 November 2014.

6   Resuscitation Council (UK) and British Heart Foundation, '2014 Guide to Automated External Defibrillators', <http://www.resus.org.uk/pages/AED_Guide.pdf>, [accessed 27 December 2014].

7   Australian Bureau of Statistics, 2013, '3303.0 – Table 1.1 Underlying cause of death, All causes, Australia', Released 31 March 2015.

8   C Lucas, 'How low can we go?', Sydney Morning Herald, 10 July 2009, <http://www.smh.com.au/national/how-low-can-we-go-20090709-depn.html>, [accessed 29 December 2014].

9   Australian Government, Bureau of Infrastructure, Transport and Regional Economics (BITRE), 'Road Trauma Australia—Annual Summaries', <https://bitre.gov.au/publications/ongoing/road_deaths_australia_annual_summaries.aspx>, [accessed 01 September 2015].

10   UK Department for Communities and Local Government, 'Fire Statistics Monitor: England April 2014 to March 2015', 2015, [online], <https://www.gov.uk/government/uploads/system/uploads/attachment_data/file/456623/Fire_Statistics_Monitor_April_2014_to_March_2015_Updated260815.pdf>, [accessed 02 September 2015].

11   BHF, Resuscitation Council (UK), NHS, ' Consensus Paper on Out-of-Hospital Cardiac Arrest in England', 16 October 2014, <https://www.resus.org.uk/pages/OHCA_consensus_paper.pdf>.

12   Australian Bureau of Statistics, 2013, loc,cit

13   FAQs 'What are my obligations? Do I need to have a fire extinguisher in my premises?', Fire Systems Services, <http://www.firesys.com.au/frequently-ask-questions-pg14873.html>..

14　'Position Statement–Selection of Residential Smoke Alarms', Fire Protection Association Australia, May 2011, Version 1.1, <http://www.fpaa.com.au/media/139827/fpa_australia_-_ps_01_v1.1_selection_of_residential_smoke_alarms.pdf>.

15　P Gourtsoyannis, 'Learn how to use defibrillator and save lives', Edinburgh Evening News, 30 July 2014, <http://www.edinburghnews.scotsman.com/life-style/learn-how-to-use-defibrillator-and-save-lives-1-3492947>, [accessed 06 April 2015].

16　ibid

17　D Gantly, 'Defribrillators (sic) are key for sudden cardiac arrests', Irish Medical Times, 10 December 2014, <http://www.imt.ie/news/latest-news/2014/12/defribrillators-key-sudden-cardiac-arrests.html>, [accessed 6 April 2015].

18　'Cancer in Australia: an overview', (2014), Australian Institute of Health and Welfare, Cancer series no. 78. Cat. no. CAN 75. Canberra: AIHW cited in Australian Government Breast Cancer webpage.
<http://canceraustralia.gov.au/affected-cancer/cancer-types/breast-cancer/breast-cancer-statistics#fn1>.

19　Australian Bureau of Statistics, 2013, loc.cit.

20　E Stromgren 'Hollywood executive's family sues gym; Alleges defibrillator negligence in death', Club Industry, 14 May 2015, [online], <http://clubindustry.com/profits/hollywood-executives-family-sues-gym-alleges-defibrillator-negligence-death>, [accessed 30 June 2015].

21　Safe Work Australia, (2012), 'Model Code of Practice – First Aid in the Workplace – Safe Work Australia', P 10, [online], <http://www.safeworkaustralia.gov.au/sites/SWA/about/Publications/Documents/693/first-aid-in-workplace.pdf > [Accessed: 30 June 2015]..

22　J Dietrich, J M Eickhoff-Shemek, C Finch, P Keyzer, K Norton, & B Sekendiz, 2014, 'The Australian Fitness Industry Risk Management Manual', Fitness Australia, Retrieved from <http://www.fitness.org.au>, <http://www.fitnessriskmanagement.com.au/pdf/The-Australian-Fitness-Industry-Risk-Management-Manual.pdf>, [Accessed 29 December 2014]; B Sekendiz, & S P Quick, 'Use of automated external defibrillators (AEDs) in managing risk and liability in health/fitness facilities', International Journal of Sport Management and Marketing 2011 9(3/4), pp. 170–184; B Sekendiz, G Gass, K Norton & C F Finch, 'Cardiac emergency preparedness in health/fitness facilities in Australia', The Physician and Sports Medicine (2014), 42(4), pp. 14–19.

23　ibid

24　ibid

25　ibid

26　AAP staff writer, 'SA coroner wants defibrillator training', The Courier Mail, 12 July 2012, <http://www.couriermail.com.au/ipad/sa-coroner-wants-defibrillator-training/story-fn6ck4a4-1226423675771>, [accessed 03 January 2015].

27　Asda Media Centre Press Release, 'Asda becomes first retailer to roll out defibs', 5 March 2014, <http://your.asda.com/press-centre/asda-becomes-first-retailer-to-roll-out-defibs>, [accessed 14 November 2014].

28　ibid

29　ibid; H Newman, 'UK | ASDA stores deploy AEDs across the nation', Big Medicine, [online] 1 October 2014, <http://bigmedicine.ca/wordpress/2014/10/uk-asda-stores-deploy-aeds-across-the-nation/#sthash.C1szTs30.dpbs>, [accessed 30 October 2014];

30　Asda Media Centre Press Release, loc.cit.

31　H Newman, loc.cit.; Asda Media Centre Press Release, loc. cit.

32   J Madaffer, Automated External Defibrillators—Deploying Slowly, OH&S Online, 1 February 2015, <http://ohsonline.com/Articles/2015/02/01/Automated-External-Defibrillators-Deploying-Slowly.aspx?admgarea=news&Page=1>.

33   Australian Bureau of Statistics, loc.cit.

34   'AHA Releases 2015 Heart and Stroke Statistics', AHA Circulation, 30 December 2014, cited on Sudden Cardiac Arrest Foundation website, <http://www.sca-aware.org/print/sca-news/aha-releases-2015-heart-and-stroke-statistics>, [accessed 5 April 2015].

35   ibid

36   US Department of Health and Human Services, National Heart, Lung, and Blood Institute, 'What Is Long QT Syndrome?', 21 September 2011, <http://www.nhlbi.nih.gov/health/health-topics/topics/qt>.

37   Commotio Cordis, <http://en.wikipedia.org/wiki/Commotio_cordi>.

38   Sudden Cardiac Arrest Foundation, 'What causes Sudden Cardiac Arrest in the Young?', [online], <http://www.sca-aware.org/sudden-cardiac-arrest-faqs>.

39   Sudden Cardiac Arrest Foundation, 'How can SCA be prevented?', [online],; <http://www.sca-aware.org/sudden-cardiac-arrest-faqs>.

40   European Society of Cardiology cited in Sudden Cardiac Arrest Foundation, 'Increase in Number of AEDs Leads to Improved Survival', 02 September 2015, [online], <http://www.sca-aware.org/sca-news/increase-in-number-of-aeds-leads-to-improved-survival>, [accessed 4 September 2015].

41   J Hansen, 'NRL and AFL support campaign to get defibrillators at all sports fields in NSW', The Sunday Telegraph, 21 June 2015, [online], <http://www.dailytelegraph.com.au/news/nsw/nrl-and-afl-support-campaign-to-get-defibrillators-at-all-sports-fields-in-nsw/story-fni0cx12-1227406337571>, [accessed 21 June 2015].

42   B Gurra, 'Emergency services in Tasmania join forces to help heart attack victims', ABC, 7 July 2015, <http://www.abc.net.au/news/2015-07-07/emergency-services-tas-join-forces-help-heart-attack-victims/660249>, [accessed 8 July 2015].

43   C Sayre, 'Saving Athletes from Cardiac Arrest', TIME Magazine, 07 May 2007, [online}, <http://content.time.com/time/health/article/0,8599,1618058,00.html>, [accessed 5 January 2015].

44   M Betts, 'Victorian sporting clubs to get heart starters', Herald Sun, 22 February 2012, <http://www.heraldsun.com.au/news/victoria/victorian-sporting-clubs-to-get-heart-starters>, [accessed 5 March 2013].

45   Baker IDI Heart & Diabetes Institute, 'Preventive Screening of Sudden Cardiac Death in Young Athletes in Australia', 25 November 2014, <https://www.bakeridi.edu.au/Suddencardiacdeath/>, [accessed 28 March 2015].

46   G McArthur, 'Carlton AFL players' heart checks assess cardiac death risk', Herald Sun, 25 November 2014, <http://www.heraldsun.com.au/news/victoria/carlton-afl-players-heart-checks-assess-cardiac-death-risk/story-fni0fit3-1227134571109?sv=3c1bc02b6a3 5e802d972b8ef10d88fe6#.VHUEftIledA.twitter>.

47   Baker IDI Heart & Diabetes Institute, loc.cit.

48   M Colquhoun, Editor, Resuscitation Council (UK) and British Heart Foundation, 'A guide to Automated External Defibrillators (AEDs)', 17 December 2013, <https://www.bhf.org.uk/~/media/files/hcps/aed_guide_final-17_12_13.pdf>, [accessed 12 April 2015].

49   M Lijovic, S Bernard, Z Nehme, T Walker and K Smith, 'Victorian Ambulance Cardiac Arrest Registry – Annual Report 2013-2014', Ambulance Victoria, <http://www.

ambulance.vic.gov.au/Media/docs/vacar-annual-report201314-25b1122a-878b-49d0-95f5-b9f10f580938-0.pdf>, [accessed 28 December 2014].

50 ibid

51 M Colquhoun, op.cit,

52 Resuscitation Central, 'History and Science of Defibrillation', <http://www.resuscitationcentral.com/defibrillation/history-science/>, [accessed 2 June 2014].

53 LA Brewer, Sphygmology through the centuries. *American Journal of Surgery*, 1920;145(6):696-702 cited in S Chihrin, *The Birth of Defibrillation: A Slow March Towards Treating Sudden Death*, University of Ontario Medical Journal, 2008 Vol 78, No 1, <http://www.uwomj.com/wp-content/uploads/2013/06/v78n1.86-90.pdf>, [accessed 25 March 2015].

54 LJ Acierno, History of Cardiology, London: The Parthenon Publishing Group, 1994 cited in S Chihrin, *The History of Defibrillation*.

55 TE Driscol, OD Ratnoff and OF Nygaard, The Remarkable Dr. Abilgaard and Countershock, Annals of Internal Medicine, 1975;83:878-882 cited in S Chihrin, *The History of Defibrillation*.

56 R Bing, *Cardiology: The Evolution of the Science and the Art*, Philadelphia: Harwood Academic Publishers, 1992 cited in S Chihrin, *The History of Defibrillation*.

57 M Peck, 'Johns Hopkins Celebrates 50 Years of CPR: The Story of Drs. Kouwenhoven, Jude and Knickerbocker', EMS Museum, 16 August 16, 22011 (revised), <http://www.emsmuseum.org/print.asp?act=print&vid=399789&section_url=by_era/>,[accessed 12 January 2015].

58 'HeartSine: A lifesaving legacy in cardiac defibrillators and mobile defibrillation technology', 1960s; <http://heartsine.com/about/our-company/history-of-innovation/>, [accessed 03 October 2014].

59 ibid

60 M Starr, 'Ambulance drone unveiled in Netherlands', EMS 1, 29 October 2014, <www.ems1.com/technology/articles/2011247-Ambulance-drone-unveiled-in-Netherlands/> [accessed 10 July 2015].

61 B Wang, 'Network of defibrillator drones could boost heart attack survival from 8% to 80%', Next Big Future, 30 October 2014, <http://nextbigfuture.com/2014/10/network-of-defibrillator-drones-could.html>, [accessed 31 October 2014].

62 L Husten, 'Grad Student Invents Flying Ambulance Drone To Deliver Emergency Shocks', Forbes,29 October 2014, <http://www.forbes.com/sites/larryhusten/2014/10/29/grad-student-invents-flying-ambulance-drone-to-deliver-emergency-shocks/>, [accessed 9 November 2014].

63 Sudden Cardiac Arrest Foundation, 'What is the difference between AEDs and defibrillators commonly used on ambulances and in hospitals?', <http://www.sca-aware.org/sudden-cardiac-arrest-faqs>.

64 M Colquhoun, op.cit.

65 Media Release, State Government of Victoria, 'Victoria's world-best cardiac survival confirmed', 7 February 2014, <https://about.myelectorate.com.au/content/victoria%E2%80%99s-world-best-cardiac-survival-confirmed>, [accessed 9 February 2014].

66 M Lijovic, S Bernard, Z Nehme, T Walker and K Smith, op.cit.

67 ibid

68   ibid

69   M Blom & S Beesems et al, 'Improved Survival After Out-of-Hospital Cardiac Arrest and Use of Automated External Defibrillators', AHA Journal, Circulation, 18 November 2014, <http://m.circ.ahajournals.org/content/130/21/1868.long>, [accessed 4 April 2015].

70   ibid

71   European Automated External Defibrillators (AED) Market Worth $134.2 Million by 2019, PRNewswire ,Fort Worth, Texas, 24 February 2015, [online] <http://www. prnewswire.com/news-releases/european-automated-external-defibrillators-aed-market-worth-1342-million-by-2019-293816081.html> [accessed 25 February 2015].

72   Madaffer, loc.cit.

73   Australian Standard AS1851:2012, 'Routine Service of Fire Protection Systems and Equipment'.

74   National Heart Foundation of Australia, Media Release, 'Heart Foundation welcomes plan to provide defibrillators to sporting clubs', 16 August 2014, <http://www. heartfoundation.org.au/news-media/Media-Releases-2014/Pages/heart-foundation-welcomes-plan-provide-defibrillators-sporting-clubs.aspx>.

75   Resuscitation Council (UK) Resuscitation Guidelines 2010, 'The use of Automated External Defibrillators', P29, <http://www.resus.org.uk/pages/aed.pdf>, [accessed 27 December 2014].

76   Traditional responders are paramedics, firefighters, police officers and first responder groups.

77   Safe Work Australia, (2012), 'Model Code of Practice – First Aid in the Workplace – Safe Work Australia', P 10, [online] Retrieved from: < http://www.safeworkaustralia.gov.au/ sites/SWA/about/Publications/Documents/693/first-aid-in-workplace.pdf > [accessed 30 June 2015].

78   National Heart Foundation of Australia, 'Heart Attack Facts – Warning signs of heart attack', <http://www.heartfoundation.org.au/driving-change/warning-signs-heart-attack/Pages/welcome.aspx>, [accessed 10 January 2015].

79   Australian Bureau of Statistics. Causes of Death data. Canberra 2012.

80   National Heart Foundation of Australia, 'Heart Attack Facts – Getting the facts on women and heart attacks', http://www.heartattackfacts.org.au/heart-attack-facts/ women-and-heart-attack/>, [accessed 10 January 2015].

81   National Heart Foundation of Australia, 'Heart Attack Facts – Warning signs of heart attack', loc.cit.

82   Resuscitation Council (UK) and British Heart Foundation, '2014 Guide to Automated External Defibrillators', op.cit.

83   Lowry v Mayo Newhall Hospital 64 ALR 4th 1191, 1196 (Cal 1986) and Board of Fire Commissioners v Ardouin (1961) 109 CLR 105, 115 as cited in M Eburn, Australian Journal of Emergency Management,'Protecting Volunteers?', Vol 18, No 4; November 2003, <https://www.em.gov.au/Documents/Protecting%20Volunteers.pdf>, [accessed 23 February 2013].

84   S Bird, 'Good Samaritans', Australian Family Physician, Vol. 37, No. 7, 2 July 2008 571, <http://www.racgp.org.au/afpbackissues/2008/200807/200807bird.pdf>, [accessed 28/01/2013].

85   K Wright, 'New law reduces delays in lifesaving care, supporters say', Dayton Daily News, 30 December 2014, <http://www.daytondailynews.com/news/news/local/new-law-reduces-delays-in-lifesaving-care-supporte/njccZ/>, [accessed 31 December 2014].

86   Ontario, Canada, Statutes and Regulations, Chase McEachern Act (Heart Defibrillator Civil Liability), 2007, <http://www.canlii.org/en/on/laws/stat/so-2007-c-10-sch-n/latest/so-2007-c-10-sch-n.html>.

87   Eburn, 'Protecting Volunteers?', loc,cit.

88   D Ipp, P Cane, D Sheldon and I Macintosh, 2002, Review of the Law of Negligence Final Report, Commonwealth of Australia, Canberra, p. 107, <http://www.amatas.com.au/assets/ipp_report.pdf>.

89   Eburn, 'Protecting Volunteers?' loc.cit.

90   S Bird, 'Good Samaritans', loc.cit.

91   M Eburn, Australian Emergency Law, [blog post], 22 March 2014, <https://emergencylaw.wordpress.com/2014/03/22/nurses-as-good-samaritans/>, [accessed 3 April 2105].

92   2014 Bondi Rescue, 'Heart Attack-Cardiac Arrest-CPR', Season 9, Ep 9, Part 1, Bondi Rescue YouTube channel, <https://www.youtube.com/watch?v=CcqfI9jRbSE>

93   Resuscitation Council (UK) Resuscitation Guidelines 2010, 'The use of Automated External Defibrillators', op.cit. P29,

94   M Lijovic, S Bernard, Z Nehme, T Walker and K Smith, op.cit.

95   Blom & Beesems et al, op.cit,.lo

96   Lijovic, Bernard, Nehme, Walker and Smith, op.cit.

97   Sudden Cardiac Arrest Foundation, AHA Releases 2015 Heart and Stroke Statistics, 30 December 2014, http://www.sca-aware.org/print/sca-news/aha-releases-2015-heart-and-stroke-statistics, [accessed 5 April 2015].

98   ibid

99   Resuscitation Council (UK) Resuscitation Guidelines 2010, 'The use of Automated External Defibrillators', op,cit,

100 K Wright, 'New law reduces delays in lifesaving care, supporters say', Dayton Daily News, 30 December 2014, <http://www.daytondailynews.com/news/news/local/new-law-reduces-delays-in-lifesaving-care-supporte/njccZ/> , [accessed 31 December 2014].

101 F Wrigley, 'Man revives woman with AED, branded a "pervert" for removing her clothes to apply electrode pads', Rocket News 24, 22 October 2014, <http://en.rocketnews24.com/2014/10/22/man-revives-woman-with-aed-branded-a-pervert-for-removing-her-clothes-to-apply-electrode-pads/>, [accessed 23 October 2014].

102 Safe Work Australia, (2012), 'Model Code of Practice, loc.cit.- P 10,

103 Wright, loc.cit.

104 Australian Bureau of Statistics, loc.cit.

105 Dietrich, Eickhoff-Shemek, Finch, Keyzer, Norton, & Sekendiz, 2014, The Australian Fitness Industry Risk Management Manual, op.cit.

106 Australian Government, How to call Triple Zero (000), <http://www.triplezero.gov.au/Documents/TripleZeroFactSheet.pdf>.

107 P Morley, Chair ARC, 2015 Spark of Life Conference cited in 'Cardiopulmonary Resuscitation Quality: Improving Cardiac Resuscitation Outcomes Both Inside and Outside the Hospital: A Consensus Statement from American Heart Association',

Circulation, 23 July 2013, pp 128:417-435, <http://circ.ahajournals.org/content/128/4/417.full.pdf+html?sid=5d6c797e-e914-4c42-b505-e6c6f44e1960>.

108 P Meaney et al, Cardiopulmonary Resuscitation Quality: Improving Cardiac Resuscitation Outcomes Both Inside and Outside the Hospital: A Consensus Statement from American Heart Association.

109 ibid

110 Resuscitation Council (UK) Resuscitation Guidelines 2010, 'The use of Automated External Defibrillators', op.cit.

111 T Murthy & B Hooda, 'Cardio Cerebral Resuscitation: Is it better than CPR?', Indian Journal of Anaesthesia, December 2009, <http://www.ncbi.nlm.nih.gov/pmc/articles/PMC2900071/> cited in: M Tesser, Emergency Live, <http://www.emergency-live.com/en/health-and-safety/cardio-cerebral-resuscitation-better-cpr?lang=en>, [accessed 12 April 2015].

112 British Heart Foundation, 'Vinnie Jones Hands-only CPR video', 4 January 2012, <https://www.youtube.com/watch?v=3vXPo7lNYzk>.

113 Murthy & Hooda, loc.cit.

114 Lijovic, Bernard, ZNehme, Walker and Smith, op.cit.

115 K Tsujimura, Programs underway to increase use of AEDs in Japan, Japan Times, 25 August 2014, <http://www.japantimes.co.jp/news/2014/08/25/national/programs-underway-to-increase-use-of-aeds-in-japan/#.Vf0C0pffuJ8>

116 BHF, Resuscitation Council (UK), NHS, 'Consensus Paper on Out-of-Hospital Cardiac Arrest in England; 16 October 2014, <https://www.resus.org.uk/pages/OHCA_consensus_paper.pdf>, [accessed 28 December 2014].

117 Resuscitation Council (UK) Resuscitation Guidelines 2010, The use of Automated External Defibrillators, op.cit.

118 ibid

119 K Navarro, 'How electrode placement affects ECGs', EMS1, 30 December 2014, <http://www.ems1.com/ecg/articles/2048422-How-electrode-placement-affects-ECGs/>, [accessed 30 December 2014].

BIBLIOGRAPHY

E Ackerman, 'The Defibrillator Drone Is Another Good Drone Idea But Will It Work?', *Spectrum*, 30 October 2014, <http://spectrum.ieee.org/automaton/robotics/aerial-robots/defibrillator-drone-another-good-drone-idea>, 9 November 2014.

M Blom & S Beesems et al, 'Improved Survival After Out-of-Hospital Cardiac Arrest and Use of Automated External Defibrillators', *Circulation, AHA Journal*, 18 November 2014, <http://m.circ.ahajournals.org/content/130/21/1868.long>.

M Link et al,' 2010 American Heart Association Guidelines for Cardiopulmonary Resuscitation and Emergency Cardiovascular Care Science', *Circulation, AHA Journal,* Part 6: Electrical Therapies, <http://circ.ahajournals.org/content/122/18_suppl_3/S706.full>.

B Lown & P Axelrod, 'Implanted Standby Defibrillators', *Circulation, AHA Journal,* 1972;46:637-639, doi:10.1161/01.CIR.46.4.637, <http://circ.ahajournals.org>.

V Menon, Two studies find bystander CPR, defibrillation linked to improved outcomes, Healio Cardiology Today, 22 July 2015, <http://www.healio.com/cardiology/arrhythmia-disorders/news/online/%7B35374234-c29f-48d4-b280-5f034c341899%7D/two-studies-find-bystander-cpr-defibrillation-linked-to-improved-outcomes>.

R J Myerburg, Editorial, 'Initiatives for Improving Out-of-Hospital Cardiac Arrest Outcomes', *American Heart Association*, Issue 21, Volume 130, November 18, 2014, <http://m.circ.ahajournals.org/content/130/21/1840>.

G Nichol et al, Editorial, 'Treatment for Out-of-Hospital Cardiac Arrest – Is the Glass Half Empty or Half Full?', *Circulation, AHA Journal,* Issue 21, Vol 130, 18 November 2014, <http://m.circ.ahajournals.org/content/130/21/1844>.

M Silverman & WB Fye, 'Profiles in Cardiology – John A. MacWilliam: Scottish Pioneer of Cardiac Electrophysiology', *Clinical Cardiology*, Vol 29, 90–92, 05 December 2006, [online], <http://onlinelibrary.wiley.com/doi/10.1002/clc.4960290213/pdf>, [accessed 10 July 2015].

K Tsujimura, Programs underway to increase use of AEDs in Japan, Japan Times, 25 August 2014, <http://www.japantimes.co.jp/news/2014/08/25/national/programs-underway-to-increase-use-of-aeds-in-japan/#.Vf0C0pffuJ8>.

'AHA Releases 2015 Heart and Stroke Statistics', 30 December 2014, *AHA Circulation*, cited on Sudden Cardiac Arrest Foundation website, <http://www.sca-aware.org/print/sca-news/aha-releases-2015-heart-and-stroke-statistics> [accessed 5 April 2015]

Defibrillation; <http://www.britannica.com/topic/defibrillation>.

External Defibrillator, How Products are Made, <http://www.madehow.com/Volume-7/External-Defibrillator.html>.

King County claims highest cardiac arrest survival rate, 20 May 2014, *My Local Health Guide.com*, <http://mylocalhealthguide.com/2014/05/20/king-county-claims-highest-cardiac-arrest-survival-rate/>.

'Pioneers in Cardiology: Frank Pantridge', CBE, MC, MD, FRCP, FACC, *AHA Circulation*, 18 December 2007, <circ.ahajournals.orgcontent11625F145.full.pdf>.

Printed in Australia
AUOC01n1219051015
270711AU00007B/21/P